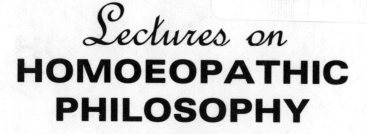

Lectures on
HOMOEOPATHIC
PHILOSOPHY

... WITH CLASSROOM NOTES ...
... AND WORD INDEX ...

JAMES TYLER KENT
A.M., M.D.

Author of Repertory of the Homoeopathic Materia Medica, and Lectures on
Homoeopathic Materia Medica, etc. Dean of the Post Graduate School of
Homoeopathy in Philadelphia for nine years. Professor of materia medica at
Hahnemann Medical College and Hospital in Chicago for six years, and of the
Herring Medical College in Chicago for some years after.

Classroom Notes Compiled
by

Dr. Harsh Nigam
M.B.B.S., M.D., M.F. (Hom.)

Seventh Edition

B. Jain Publishers (P) Ltd.
An ISO 9001: 2000 Certified Company
USA – Europe – India

LECTURES ON HOMOEOPATHIC PHILOSOPHY WITH CLASSROOM NOTES AND WORD INDEX

Seventh Edition: 2007
Reprint Edition: 2009

Published by Kuldeep Jain for
B. JAIN PUBLISHERS (P) LTD.
An ISO 9001 : 2000 Certified Company
1921/10, Chuna Mandi, Paharganj, New Delhi 110 055 (INDIA)
Tel.: 91-11-2358 0800, 2358 1100, 2358 1300, 2358 3100
Fax: 91-11-2358 0471 • *Email:* info@bjain.com
Website: **www.bjainbooks.com**

Printed in India by
J.J. Offset Printers

ISBN: 978-81-319-0260-8

Contents

Publisher 's Note to Seventh Edition

B. JAIN Publishers (P) Ltd. is relentlessly working in the field of homoeopathy since a long time and trying its best to provide antique literature in the best possible user friendly form. Thus, the 7th edition of the "Lectures on Homoeopathic Philosophy" by J. T. Kent is available in the reader's hands.

Immense care has been taken while editing the book regarding the matter concerned in each lecture.

New eye-catchy look has been provided to each lecture and aphorisms have been properly highlighted.

Word index at the end of the book will help the reader to catch hold of related matter or topic at a glance.

It is expected that readers will fully avail this historic literature of J.T. Kent.

In addition, without moving the original philosophy, an easy explanation to lectures is added by Dr. Harsh Nigam at the close of original literature so that readers can have thorough understanding of Master's philosophy. We appreciate Dr. Harsh Nigam for his earnest efforts.

Kuldeep Jain
MD, B. Jain Publishers

Publisher's Note to Sixth Edition

B. JAIN Publishers (P) Ltd. is relentlessly working in the field of homoeopathy since a long time and trying its best to provide antique literature in the best possible user friendly form. Thus, the 6ᵗʰ edition of the "Lectures on Homoeopathic Philosophy" by J. T. Kent is available in the reader's hands.

Immense care has been taken while editing the book regarding the matter concerned in each lecture.

New eye-catchy look has been provided to each lecture and aphorisms have been properly highlighted.

Word index at the end of the book will help the reader to catch hold of related matter or topic at a glance.

It is expected that readers will fully avail this historic literature of J.T. Kent.

Kuldeep Jain
MD, B. Jain Publishers

Foreword to Classroom Notes

THIS BOOK is written for those who feel difficulty in understanding the background of Kent's philosophy and his basic approach towards Hahnemann.

Without through knowledge of Kent's philosophy, Homeopathic practice is senseless, irrational and like a living body without soul.

For any good and right prescriber a grasp of basic principle of Homeopathy is necessary and this can be learned by only two books:

1. Hahnemann's Organon.
2. Kent's philosophy.

Ever since Hahnemann has written the Organon no Homeopath is exempted from the obligation to transcribe a complete case history. As Hahnemann has mentioned no remedy is simillimum unless it contains the sum and essence of morbid symptoms.

Hahnemann directs us to pay most of our attention to the symptoms of the mind, because the symptoms of the mind constitute the person himself. The highest and innermost symptoms are the mind symptoms. Irritability and mental depression run through a great many remedies and these form the center around which all the mental symptoms revolve in so many cases these days.

The mentals can be classified in a person. The things that relate to the memory are not so important as the things that relate to the intelligence. The things that relate to the intelligence are not so important as the things that relate to the affections.

We see that in the state of irritability the patient is not irritable while doing the things that he desires to do. If he wants to be talked to, for instance, you do not discover his irritability while talking to him. Just as you do something that he doesn't like, this irritability or the disturbance of will is brought on, and this reflects the innermost of the individual's state. The things that he wishes belong to the will and therefore the things that belong to the will are the most important things in the provings.

Put it this way—if an individual is sad, why is he sad? Is it because he lacks something that he wants? This sadness may go on to such an extent that the mind is in confusion. Confusion of mind due to sadness and the confusion of mind due to vertigo are two different things. One must make distinction. Vertigo is not a confusion of intelligence. One has to ponder upon it for a moment. Confusion of mind is a disturbance of intellect and not a disturbance of sensorium.

These things must be thought out carefully, so that we are clear in our mind as to what symptoms mean. That is why it is important to record the language of the patient. Often a patient will say something, which you can see he does not mean and then it becomes necessary for the physician to know what he really means.

For instance a female patient says — "I have such a pain in my chest" with hands on the abdomen around menses. You know it may be a painful uterus. Now it is your duty to ascertain whether the pain is really in the chest or the patient, due to her shyness is not telling you the right thing.

You must understand that an individual's intellectual nature keeps the person in contact with his environment, but his emotions (affects) are largely kept to himself. A person can have affections for all sort of things and perversions of those affections, but his intellect will guide him not to show his likes and dislikes to the world. The affects cannot be seen but a person's intellect is subject to inspection. One cannot conceal intellect. We have to observe that the will (affections / emotions) are the innermost and these are covered with a cloak of understanding (intellect) just like a person wears a garment to hide his body.

According to Hahnemann, the so-called mental and emotional diseases are only organic diseases, in which mental disturbances are aggravated while the physical symptoms diminish. Hahnemann does not accept that there is an autonomous psychic life separate from physical bodily processes. He considers neurosis as a functional derangement of whole person.

Neurosis and physical disease are two expression of a disease process that begins with disturbance in the vital plane.

Dr. Harsh Nigam has tried to present Kent's philosophy in his own structured style. I believe and hope that the students of Homeopathic school and the novice Homeopathist will enjoy reading this book written with a definite clear vision and honest intention.

Dr. Jagdish Chandra Nigam

37/51, Gilis Bazar
Kanpur, India

Preface to Classsroom Notes

STUDY of Kentain thought in Homeopathy is essential to a beginner at some stage because Kent understood and discerned between the science and the art, as he could discren medicine from spirituality (religion). These two like many other things in this universe appear paradoxical, but in reality they are two sides of the same coin. You master one and the second one slowly opens to you. To the students I say understand and perceive Kent and to the exponents I request revisit Kent with an open mind and sophisticated thinking.

The original relationship between religion and science has been of integration and this integration is clearly seen in eastern medical philosophy of Ayurveda and Chinese medicine. Greek thinkers like Plato, Aristotle and Aquinas are of the same line of thought.

In the 16th century, however the relationship between science and regligion began to go sour and hit rock bottom in 1633 when Galilio was summoned before inquisition.

In response to this trend there emerged toward the end of the 17th and the beginning of the 18th century, an unwritten social contract that divided the territory between government, science and religion.

In some ways this unwritten social contract might be looked upon as one of the great intellectual happenings of human kind. All kind of good came from it. The inquisition faded away, religious folk stopped burning witches, the coffers of the church remained full for several centuries, slavery was abolished, democracy was established without anarchy, and although science restricted itself to natural phenomenon, science thrived, giving birth to a technological revolution beyond anybody's wildest expectations.

Although not consciously developed this unwritten social contract was almost a spontaneous response to the need of the day and it had done, more than anything else to determine the nature of our science and our religion ever since.

There was a minority at that time which was exploring new ways beyond the science of the day and men like Samuel Hahnemann were experimenting with non-material forces to treat disease phenomenon. One other contemporary of note was Mesmer, who was exploring the forces of mind (primitive psychology).

In early 1700's, Sir Isaac Newton, then the president of Royal Society of London for improving natural knowledge devised a contract, which distinguished Natural Knowledge from Para-natural Knowledge (Occult/ Mysticism).

Natural knowledge had become the province of science, while the occult became the province of religion, and one effect of that separation was the emasculation of philosophy but for one Samuel Hahnemann who was a true philosopher in the lines of Aristotle, Socrates, Francis Bacon.

Now the problem is, that this unwritten social contract no longer works. Indeed, at this point of time, it is becoming diabolic, the word diabolic comes from the Greek diaballein, which means to throw apart or to separate, to comparatmentalize. It is the opposite of "symbolic", which comes from the word of symballein, meaning to throw together, unify.

Medicine today although technologically superb and suave, it is comparatmentalizing patients and this model of super-specialization is not working. We as Homeopaths belong to the holistic model of medicine.

Looking back over the course of human history, we can discern both the strengths and the limitations inherent in the age of faith. Only recently we are beginning to see the limitations of the age of reason, which is were we now find ourselves as a society.

I have often wondered what might be beyond this age of reason. I do not know. I hope it will be the age of integration. In that age natural knowledge and so called occult knowledge will work hand in had and both will be more sophisticated as result.

Before we can arrive at the age of integration we ourselves must become more sophisticated in our thinking. Specifically, we must learn how to think paradocixally because we will encounter paradox whenever reason becomes integrated with experience/ faith.

That is the reason I would like to invoke Kent because in Homeopathy, Kent was a blend of science, reason, experience and faith. I have added three new chapters, on repertorisation, on prescribing and on trend of thought necessary for development in Homeopathy, none of the words are mine. It is all written by Kent in his minor writing. My job has been to arrange diverse writings under singular heading.

This book is an attempt to present the core of science, art and philosophy of true Homeopathy in a modern way, debulking it for the sake of the modern reader but I would urge serious exponents of Homeopathy to go through the original text by Kent.

I am thankful to Dr. Harpreet Kaur for editorial assistance and above all to Mr. Kuldeep Jain of B. Jain Publisher because of whom this small work finds its place at the feet of Master Kent in the form of Classroom Notes.

Dr. Harsh Nigam

Preface by

Dr. Kent

THESE LECTURES were delivered in the POST GRADUATE SCHOOL OF HOMOEOPATHICS, and published in the Journal of Homoeopathics, and, now in somewhat revised form, are given to the profession with the hope that they will prove useful to some in giving a clearer apprehension of the doctrines of Homoeopathy. They are not intended, in any sense, to take the place of the Organon, but should be read with that work, in the form of a commentary, the object in each lecture being to dwell upon the particular doctrine sufficiently to perceive and emphasize the master's thought. Not all of the paragraphs in the Organon have been considered, as many of them are sufficiently clear to the reader and their teaching is quite obvious.

Homoeopathy is now extensively disseminated over the world, but, strange to say, by none are its doctrines so distorted as by many of its pretended devotees. Homoeopathics treats of both the science and the art of healing by the law of similars, and if the art is to remain and progress among men the science must be better understood than at present. To apply the art without the science is merely a pretension, and such practice should be relegated to the domain of empiricism. To safely practice the art of curing sick people, the homoeopathic physician must know the science.

It is not expected that this course of lectures covers the whole field of homoeopathic philosophy, but it is intended to serve as an introduction to further study, and as a text-book for students, that they may have a sound starting, and become interested in the objects of this work.

James Tyler Kent

Evanston, Ill, July 1, 1900

Publisher's Preface

Fifth Edition

"**KENT STILL** lives! His influence still shines as a burning torch to reveal truth!"

From the far corners of the earth, Pakistan, India, South America, Mexico, everywhere comes proof of that prophecy . . . the coming generation is demanding the messages of the master, the master who scaled the heights of the Homoeopathic Law of Cure.

A revival of faith and new adherents everywhere make Kent's books more and more sought after and we herewith present to the profession the fifth edition of the Philosophy in full knowledge that it will fulfill its great mission for the present and the future generations as it has in the past.

In as much as all four previous editions have been exhausted this fifth edition will be hailed far and wide with eager desire . . . which we, the publishers, and glad to have the power to fulfill.

Ehrahart & Karl
Publishers
Chicago, July 1954

James Tyler Kent

An Appreciation

by

A. Eugene Austin, M.D., H.M.

Hail Kent !

Prometheus-like, thy flame so bright.
Has brought to us a ray to light
From Hahnemann's shining path, so fond
It blazes wondrous realms beyond
Health, for poor groping human-kind,
A paradise on earth will find.
Dead? No! Thy living law, its seeds will sow
That good, diffused, may more abundant grow.
Hail Kent!

CAN ANYONE say "Kent is dead!" Kent is laid away amid the snow-capped mountains of Montana!"

Kent never died! The earthly shrine of his immortal mind returns to dust amid the western mountains-Kent still lives.

Kent's intense desire to alleviate suffering, to eradicate disease led him to concentrate, by the power of his indomitable will, the forces of his vast intellect. He gave himself unstintingly to the arduous task of acquiring that deep knowledge by which he scaled the heights of the Homoeopathic Law of Cure. Here his unclouded vision beheld the genius of Samuel Hahnemann. He grasped the Master's thought, he wielded the healing power, he reached greater heights.

Kent was discoverer of Series and Degrees. He blazoned new paths of practical research. His keen perception selected a comparatively few of the more receptive and studious from the larger body of students of the medical colleges where he lectured that he might impart to them the deeper lore which he had through long years painstakingly acquired. These students of the privileged inner circle all but idolized their learned, beloved master. They organized themselves in November 1910, into the Society of Homoeopathicians that the master's messages might more readily reach all, and through them be disseminated by their own practice of pure Homoeopathy, and by the publication of their journal, *The Homoeopathician*. Kent's objective was like that of this society of his students, "to foster and develop the principals of Homoeopathy as *promulgated by Samuel Hahnemann,* to increase knowledge of them and of their application."

Kent worte voluminously with exactness and precision for many medical publication. His Materia Medica, Kent's Repertory and Kent's Philosophy are medical classics whose value will grow with the years. His writings are published in many languages. He has devoted followers in many nations, especially India.

Like the Seer of Cothen, Kent of America reverently and understandingly pondered God's open Books of Nature and Revelation. To God they gave the praise for all that He enabled them to do by the Divine Law, *"Similia Similibus Curantur."* Both overcame crushing trails and difficulties in the battle for truth.

O Kent, no tribute I can pay can equal the debt I owe! You sent for me. You poured your love upon me, taught me. You gave me many provileged hours in your Chicago Office; took me into closer fellowship for days and nights in your home and garden at Evanston. Later, when I was again in my office in New York, and death was drawing me away, you called me back by you skill. When physicians failed to cure, to you they brought the hopeless minds and bodies of their patients, and you healed the many. You were moved to tears when I told you how in Perela-Chaise I gratefully covered with flowers the grave of Samuel Hahnemann. O Kent, beloved friend, elder brother, physician, master, seer, let a double portion of thy spirit rest on all thy loyal followers the world over who would unite with me in laying an unfading tribute of appreciation of the choicest treasures of our heart's grateful, admiring devotion on your bier.

(The Alpha Sigma Semi-Annual, Vol 2, No. 1, May, 1917)
Through the Courtesy of the Fraternity.

Dr. James Tyler Kent

THERE ARE many men in this world of ours, but there and few masters. Among may pleasantest recollections are the moments spent at the feet, as it were, of this master of Homoeopathy.

Dr. Kent was a man of exceptionally keen observation. He knew disease with all its intricacies, its complications, its peculiarities as very few men know it. He knew the spirit of the Materica Medica as very few men had learned to know it. His remarkable genius of selecting a similimum on the plane of the disease for which he prescribed was really phenomenal almost magical. It seemed to me at times that he could give a remedy with a magical touch far exceeding that of my comprehension.

This was natural for him, and yet to his natural genius and power of concentration he added years of unstinted study. This made him one of the greatest masters in medicine the world has ever known.

May it be given to each of us to read and study this book in the spirit in which it was written, and with the same power of concentration that discovered and revealed such remarkable truths.

G.E. Dienst
February 21, 1919

Dr. James Tyler Kent

ONLY TO some is it given to attain the distinction of success along a single line of endeavour; to but a few it is permitted to lead in more than one accomplishment; while only once in a life time is an individual born who goes beyond these.

Such a man was our late master, James Tyler Kent. Fulfilling the significant *"Homoeopathic Trinity,"* he was a fearless investigator and writer; a thorough, conscientious teacher and leader, and a marvelous practitioner.

The medical profession at large will agree in the first attribute; those of us who had a privilege of his teaching and counsel will bear witness to the second; and the large number of sick people who were cured by him during his forty or more years of medical activity (many of them after others had failed), will substantiate the last.

Our school has developed many fearless investigators, a few notable teachers and quite a number of good practitionaers; but since Hahnemann only in his one man have been so brilliantly combined the three attributes that enables Homoeopathy to stand so firmly in these times of medical Nihilis.

Intolerant of sham, firm in the application of the Homoeopathic principles, and the almost uncanny in his prescience, we can well say with Shakespeare :

> "His life was gently, and the elements
> So marked in him, that Nature might stand up
> And say to all the world, this was a man."

C.P. Thacher

Dr. James Tyler Kent

DR. KENT'S work on the Philosophy of Homoeopathy ranks with the world's finest literature.

To the homoeopath it is indispensable, as it is the key that unblocks the storehouse of knowledge relative to the art of homoeopathic healing.

A full knowledge of this work clarifies many of the obscure points in the Organon and enables the physician to perceive deeper into homoeopathic truth.

To use the repertory expertly, it is necessary to have a complete knowledge of the contents of this book.

To show how to study the Material Medica in order to grasp it fully and to apply it successfully this work has no equal.

A.H. Grimmer, M.D.

Dr. James Tyler Kent

WHAT MEMORIES, or rather visions, that name calls forth! The small man, shrunken and gray when I first saw him, but giving the impression of force and clearness; the keen eyes whose direct gaze through his glasses looked you through and through; the quite strength of personality when talking of the Homoeopathy which dominated him there was no room for comment on his ill-fitting and ill assorted clothes; he ignored his clothes and his dark office in his consuming enthusiasm for his work, and his listeners ignored them too. His health was very poor after I knew him; if vigorous in early manhood he must have been a tower of strength.

Genial, gentle, devoted friend to his patients, and pupils; jealous guardian of pure Homoeopathy against the criticisms of those whom he considered his enemies; sensitive, embittered, retiring man in later years as he thought one after another did him wrong it makes us think of the experience of Hahnemann, yet I feel sure Dr. Kent had many more friends than he thought he had; most of his patients and pupils were devoted to him and he basked in the sunshine of that devotion.

Keen-minded, faithful student and philosopher, one of the few great ones since Hahnemann, where shall we find another such? He became dissatisfied with his results in allopathic prescribing; he was open minded, searcher after truth, so he followed a suggestion given to him to go and see the results in Homoeopathy; he, like others, wanted to ridicule at first, but he saw that Homoeopathy cured and straightaway set himself to learn it thoroughly; his whole life there-after was devoted with untiring enthusiasm to its study and practice.

Teacher of Homoeopathy, where shall we find another anywhere near him? A clear interpreter of the philosophy, a human touch, bringing matters which seemed hidden and complex out into the light of practical, everyday experience and yet endowing them with a reverence, a sublimity that is marvelous.

A wonderful vision of the heart and persoality of the homoeo-pathic remedies, how he could make them live to his students! Shed of encumbering detail, with all obscure characteristics made clear, these remedies become concentrate realities.

Compiler of the largest and most comprehensive homoeo-pathic repertory extant, built on easily comprehended framework and carried to infinite detail, we marvel that any one man could complete such a work. This alone would made Dr. Kent live for all time to students of Homoeopathy.

Publisher of his lectures on philosophy and Materia Medica just as he delivered them in the classroom so that they might be as vivid to every reader as to his immediate pupils; we thank him for that.

Consulting physician, with patients scattered all over the world, with nearly every practitioner of pure Homoeopathy appealing to him for help in time of trouble, and with students coming from foreign countries to be near for his counsel what a unique figure in any profession.

Is this all? No, for after all these general statements each one of Dr. Kent's pupils comes foreword with the evidence of the help he or she obtained. I am glad that he called me one of his pupils and liked to do so. I never was in his classroom, but I studied his lectures and repertory and have followed his teachings in practice. To me his way of presenting a subject is the way I can grasp that subject and use it in my work. I am sure I owe to Dr. Kent the largest share of whatever success in Homoeopathy I have achieved, for without his clear method of interpreting I should have found the road hard indeed.

And after this comes the evidence of help obtained by patients all through this country and scattered over the world. Dr. Kent cured my mother on reports alone, without ever seeing her and her condition was most obscure and alarming; he helped my father greatly for years, though his trouble was incurable; cured me of deep chronic tendencies; told me what constitutional remedy my brother needed and then bade me treat him myself, but he has never needed further treatment.

So it goes, on and on. The spirit of James Tyler Kent lives in his works, even as the spirit of Hahnemann lives in his, and many, many hearts are grateful.

Julia Minerva Green
Washington, D.C. Feb., 1919

Dr. James Tyler Kent

A **STUDY** of Doctor Kent's life and achievement reveals three prominent attributes: Rare intution of perception; logical thought and a love or order so strong that implicit obedience to law and uncompromising devotion to principle were set as his ideal as against personal interest and inclination. These qualities enabled him to recognize and acknowledge the Law of Cure and the existence and operation of the vital force or Dynamis; to explore the nature of the mental and physical disturbances we call diseases as well as the artifical diseases which we term "drug action;" and finally to apply the knowledge so gained to the cure of sickness. He was able to penetrate and unravel as few if any before have done the intricate nature and relationships of the drugs of our rich Materia Media, making distinctions as to the planes of drug action never before formulated as far as I am aware.

In the whole domain of therapeutic science he rose to untrod heights of vision, and at the same time descended to most thorough exploration of the valleys of investigation and applied knowledge; as a final result placing in the hands of his followers those volumes which for ages to come will serve as a guiding light and armamentarium for effective and precise work in healing, the "Materia Medica," the "Repertory," and this his crowning work, the "Homoeopathic Philosophy."

Such vision as his is not given except to the possessor of humility (the forerunner of wisdom); and this quality he had in common with his great teacher Hahnemann, although in both it was disguised to many by a robust and aggressive championship of the truth. The vision of both these great thinkers was clarified by a spiritual tendency of thought, which impelled them boldly to challenge a materialistic (with an authority not of human self-intelligence) reasserting the doctrine of a dual universe a world of spirit, of causes, of living forces, within the visible world of effects, of dead forces and matters. Without such a position—

without an interna active and an externa passive or reactive—
there could be no science of Homoeopathy.

For his ability to further unfold and advance the science of
Homoeopathy, Doctor Kent was confessedly indebted to another
mastermind, Emanuel Swedenborg, whose position as a scientist
and investigator is tardily being recognized by leading scientific
minds in Europe and America. With a genius that combined in
unique degree the faculties of intuition and of rational deduction,
Swdenborg brought to bear upon the problems of creation and of
the created universe certain new doctrines whereby he was able
to evolve what may well be called the "philosophy of science."
Among these were the doctrines of Series and Degrees.

Not once, by many times. Doctor Kent has said to me
substantially these words : "All my teachings is founded on that
of Hahnemann and of Swedenborg; their teachings correspond
prefectly." And also, "Truth is not of man; he is only the
imperfect vehicle of its expression." This acknowledgement of
indebtedness has been made to many of his pupils, and needs
recording here for its bearing upon both the antecedents and the
quality of his work.

Doctor Kent's work, Hahnemann's work, Swedenborg's work,
is not done; it is just in its beginning. Ages hence, when the race
shall have been delivered from the incubus of its ills, spiritual,
mental and physical, their contributions to the happy outcome
will be given a recognition beyond our power to formulate now.

_____

Goerge G. Starkey

Dr. James Tyler Kent

TO THE memory of the late Dr. James Tyler Kent nothing can be said that would, in any way, do justice to his genius and skill as a Homoeopathic physician. He was not only a physician, but above all a man, measuring up to the highest standards of morality and honesty, fully and thoroughly imbued with the highest ideals of his profession. He was, through his career as a physician, as honest, painstaking prescriber, who considered the welfare of his patient above his own pecuniary interest; this quality, added to his Homoeopathic profession, much valuable literature upon the subject of Homoeopathy in the way of text-books, covering such subjects as Materia Medica the Philosophy of Homoeopathy and his stupendous work, the Repertory. These are not ordinary publications, but are considered classics by the profession. To the student of Homoeopathy let me drop a hint, and it is this: if you wish to become proficient in the thoroughly mastered the purport of its contents. Do not think one moment that one reading will give you an understanding of the principles set forth; it will not, but will require many careful perusals until its subject matter becomes a part of yourself, then only will it be of service to you.

His utterances on Materia Medica and Repertory are the tolls which will enable you to perform your work after you have grasped the working principles contained within this valued treasure book.

Elmer Schwartz, M.D.

Dr. James Tyler Kent

I AM pleased to learn that you are to publish another edition of Dr. J.T. Kent's philosophy of Homoeopathy, a book which every true physician who is seeking the truth should not only have in this possession, but one to which he should frequently read and study its very valuable lessons.

I was closely connected with the late Dr. Kent for many years and learned to know him well. I prize very highly the memory of these years for the very valuable lessons taught to me by him. He was a master Homoeopath, always willing to help and guide the student, keeping the truth of the law a cure.

His books are now among the most valuable in the medical libraries and world over. To those who were not fortunate enough to know Doctor Kent personally, I must heartily recommend his works and hope this new edition of the Philosophy will have the wide sale it deserves.

W.W. Sherwood, M.D.

Highlights of Kent's Lectures on Homoeopathic Philosophy

THE DISCOVERY of homoeopathic philosophy brought an altogether *new era* of thoughts in the world of Practice of medicine. To understand this we have to have a look on the existing system of that time.

Introduction

✦ The old school or *Allopathy* considered about *'sickness'* and *'medicine'* in a particular way.

✦ The sphere of sickness was limited to the physical level. Only tissue changes were seen and considered.

✦ The *source* of sickness, *process* of sickness, the *nature* of sickness and the concept of real health were *not* studied.

✦ Only the result of sickness was *felt with fingers,* seen with eyes and observed by sense through *instruments*.

✦ The meaning of *restoration* of health was confined to relief in the ailments of particular *organs* where they appeared.

✦ *Drugs* were used in *crude* forms to remove the ailments.

✦ The system was based entirely on *experience*. Decisions were made on *opinions* of individuals at different times and concensus of opinions or hypothesis.

✦ Pathological findings formed the basis of the *diagnosis*.

✦ The *internal of man*—his mental and emotional aspects were not considered.

✦ *Symptoms*—the language of sickness, at the levels of mind, emotion and body were not studied.

✦ Every pathological result had its corresponding *bacteria*.

✦ Doctrine of *Vital Force* had no place for them.

✦ Prime importance was given to the *organs of man,* and not to the man himself which constituted of body mind and emotions.

✧ Will and *understanding* of man not studied and considered.

Homoeopathic Philosophy

DR. HAHNEMANN 'proved' the drugs on *healthy enlightened human bodies*. He found that the drugs affected the mind, the emotions and the body and the effects are expressed through symptoms and modalities. He also found that these drugs in potency are able to remove Similar Sickness appearing in human beings. He discovered an Universal Truth; a truth based on 'science' where opinions do not matter, experience do not form basis; source of sickness, process of sickness and the nature of sickness is explored and the *correct curative agent is found*.

Dr. Kent has interpreted and explained the various aspects of Hahnemann's "Organon of the Healing Art". His lectures are so *vivid* that they mirror the fundamental laws of health and healing to the mankind at all levels of understanding. This book was written about *90 years* ago-but still, the concepts hold true in the present times. He was an empirical Hahnemannian. He could not compromise with the deviation from principles and philosophy and we find his criticism sometimes sharp and bitter of 'Pseudo-homoeopaths'.

Keynotes of Philosophy

✧ Man is the *will and the understanding* and the house which he lives in is his body.

✧ The *organs* are not the man. The man is prior to the organs.

✧ The order of sickness as well as the order of cure is from man to his organs. The real sick man is prior to the sick body.

✧ A man is sick prior to *localizaion* of disease. When we wait for localization, the results of disease have rendered the patient incurable.

✧ Symptoms are but the *language of nature,* talking out, as it were, and showing as clearly as the daylight, the internal nature of the sickman or woman.

✧ *Crude* drugs cannot heal the sick and that what changes they effect are not real but only *apparent.*

✧ Tissue changes are of the body and are the results of the disease, they are *not the disease.*

✧ The bacteria are results of the disease. The disease cause is more subtle.

✧ The remedy, which will produce on healthy man *similar symptoms,* is the master of the situation, is the necessary antidote, will overcome the sickness, restore the will and understanding to order and cure the patient.

✧ Man consists in what he thinks and what he loves and there is nothing else in man.

✧ The physician has to 'perceive' in the disease that which is to be cured, and that is through 'totality of symptoms'. He has to perceive the nature of disease and the nature of the remedy.

✧ Experience has only a *confirmatory place.* It cannot take the place of science and truth.

✧ All true diseases of the economy flow from *centre to circumference.* All miasms are true diseases.

✧ The active cause is within, and the apparent cause of sickness is without. If a man has no deep miasmatic influence, outer causes will not affect him.

✧ Homoeopathy has two parts: the science of homoeopathy and the *art of homoeopathy.* One has to learn the art of homoeopathy to prepare himself for the application of the science of homoeopathy.

✧ *Vital force* is constructive and formative, and in its absence there is death and destruction.

✧ Every human being has his *atmosphere or aura;* every thing in the universe has its aura. Every star and planet has it. The remedy to be homoeopathic must be similar in quality and similar in action to the disease cause.

✧ As soon as the *internal economy* is deprived in any manner of its freedom, death is threatening; where freedom is lost, death is sure to follow.

- ✧ Potency should suit the varying *susceptibility* of sick man.
- ✧ Any more than just enough to supply the susceptibility is a surplus and is dangerous.
- ✧ Human race has been greatly disordered in the economy because of *surplus drug taking*.
- ✧ Primitive cause is not in the *bacteria*. Bacteria themselves have a cause to appear and survive.
- ✧ Over sensitive patients are actually poisoned by the *inappropriate administration* of potentized medicines.
- ✧ Their chronic miasms are complicated with chronic drugging and its effect upon the vital force.
- ✧ The physician who can only *hold in his memory* the symptoms of a disease or a remedy *will never succeed* as a homoeopath.
- ✧ The majority of such as call themselves homoeopaths at the present time, are perfectly incompetent to examine a patient, and therefore incompetent to examine homoeopathy.
- ✧ It is impossible to test homoeopathy without learning how to get the *disease image* so before the eyes that the homoeopathic remedy can be selected.
- ✧ At the present day, there is almost no such thing as an unprejudiced mind.
- ✧ Do not prescribe until you have found the remedy that is *similar to the whole case,* even although it is clear in your mind that one remedy may be more similar to one particular group of symptoms and another remedy to another group.
- ✧ It is unaccountable, therefore, that some of our homoeo-pathic practitioners make use of *palliatives* that are so detrimental to the patients.

Comments

DR. KENT was a philosopher and a scientist of high order in the world of medicine. He had a *dream of achievement*, an ideal to fulfil. But he was too strict and could not *anticipate* the practical aspect and the fate of science when practiced on a mass scale all over the world. During his *own time*, he could not find a sufficient number of physicians who could practice within the framework of philosophy and bring success and glory to the science. *While our great pioneer wanted a dose of a single remedy to be given after being fully satisfied with the totality of symptoms, in appropriate potency, without unrequired repetition*, we find today that people are using mixtures of various remedies without any consideration of *symptoms* on Allopathic patterns the *World Over*. The deviation is in a way downfall of homoeopathy 'the greatest Science of healing' brought to the human race by Dr. Hahnemann.

But the great pioneer has left a message and responsibility with the next generation. "While Homoeopathy itself is a perfect science, its truth is only partially known. The truth itself relates to the divine and the knowledge relates to the man. It will require a long time before physicians become genuine masters in this truth". And it is our pious duty to prepare ourselves for the capability that the science requires to bestow real health to the ailing human beings on the earth.

K.D. Kanodia
Delhi, October, 1991

A Tribute

All hail James Tyler Kent, to all endeared,
Whom, as their chief, his pupils proudly claim.
In ages yet unborn shall be revered,
By countless hosts, his never-dying name.

We, who have groped in ignorance as blind,
Rejoice as those who have received new sight;
This gift we owe to his colossal mind,
And through his teachings revel in the light.

The fire he kindled has been duly fanned
And cannot now be quenched by floods or seas;
The leaping flames spread on through every land,
Restoring health and banishing disease.

Henry B. Blunt, M.D., C.M.

LECTURE I

§ 1. "The Sick"

HOMOEOPATHY asserts that there are *principles* which govern the practice of medicine. It may be said that, up till the time of Hahnemann, no principles of medicine were recognized, and even at this day in the writings and actions of the Old Schools there is a complete acknowledgment that no principles exist. The Old School declares that the practice of medicine depends entirely upon experience, upon what can be found out by giving medicines to the sick. Their shifting methods and theories, and rapid discoveries and abandonment of the same, fully attest the sincerity of their acknowledgements and declarations. Homoeopathy leaves Allopathy at this point, and so in this manner the great division between the two schools is affected. That there are principles Homoœpathy affirms. The Old School denies the existence of principles and with apparent reason, looking at the matter from the standpoint of their practice and methods. They deal only with ultimates, they observe only results of disease, and either deny or have no knowledge of the real nature of man, what he is, where he came from, what his quality is in sickness or in health. They say nothing about the man except in connection with his tissues; they characterize the changes in the tissues as the disease and all there is of the disease, its beginning and its end. In effect they proclaim disease to be something that exists without a cause. They accept nothing but what can be felt with the fingers and seen with the eyes or otherwise observed through the sense, aided by improved instruments.

The finger is aided by the microscope to an elongated point, and the microscopic pathological results of disease are noted and considered to be the beginning and the ending, *i.e.* result without anything prior to them. That is a summary of allopathic teaching as to the nature of sickness. But Homoeopathy perceives that there is something prior to these results. Every science teaches, and every investigation of a scientific character proves that everything which exists does so because of something prior to it. Only in this way can we trace cause and effect in a series from beginning to end and back again from the end to the beginning. By this means we arrive at a state in which we do not assume, but in which we know.

The first paragraph of the *Organon* will be understood by an inexperienced observer to mean one thing and by a true and experienced homoeopath to mean another.

---

§ 1. "The physician's high and only mission is to restore the sick to health, to cure as it is termed."

No controversy will arise from a superficial reading of this statement, and until Hahnemann's hidden meaning of the world "sick" is fully brought to view, the physician of any school will assent. The idea that one person will entertain as to the meaning of the word "sick" will be different at times from that which another will entertain. So long as it remains a matter of opinion, there will be differences of opinion, therefore the homoeopath must abandon the mere expressions of opinion. Allopathy rests on individual opinion and Allopaths say that the science of medicine is based on the consensus of opinion, but that is an unworthy and unstable foundation for the science of curing the sick. It will never be possible to establish a rational system of therapeutics until we reason from facts as they are and not as they sometimes appear. Facts as they appear are expressed in the opinion of men, but facts as they are, are facts and truths from which doctrines are evolved and formulated which will interpret or unlock the kingdoms of nature in the realm of sickness or health. Therefore, beware of the opinion of men in science Hahnemann has given us principles which we can study and advance upon. It is law that governs the world and not matters of opinion or hypotheses. We must begin by having a respect for law, for we have no starting point unless we base our propositions on law. So long as we recognize men's statements we are in a state of change, for men and hypotheses change. Let us acknowledge the authority.

The true homoeopath, when he speaks of *the sick*, knows who it is that is sick, whereas the allopath does not know. The latter thinks that the house which the man lives in, which is being torn down, expresses all there is of sickness; in other words, that the tissue changes (which are only the *results* of disease) are all that there is of the sick man. The homoeopath observes wonderful changes resulting from potentized medicine, and being compelled to reflect he sees that crude drugs cannot heal the sick and that what changes they do effect are not real but only apparent. Modern physiology has no vital doctrine in its teaching, and therefore no basis to work upon. The doctrine of the vital force is not admitted by the teachers of physiology and, therefore, the homoeopath sees that true physiology is not yet taught, for without the vital force, without simple substance, without the internal as well as the external, there can be no *cause* and no relation between cause and effect.

Now what is meant by "the sick?" It is a man that is sick and to be restored to health, not his body, not the tissues. You will find many people who will say, "I am sick." They will enumerate pages of symptoms, pages of suffering. They look sick. But they tell you, "I have been to the most eminent physicians. I have had my chest examined. I have been to the neurologist. I have been to the cardiac specialist and have had my heart examined. The eye specialist has examined my eyes. I have been to the gynecologist and have had my uterus examined", says the woman. "I have been physically examined from head to foot, and they tell me I am not sick, I have no disease." Many a time have I heard this story after getting three or four pages of symptoms. What does it mean? It is true if that state progresses there will *be* evidences of disease, *i.e.,* evidences which the pathologist may discover by his physical examination. But at present the patient is not sick, says the learned doctor. "But what do all these symptoms mean? I do not sleep at night. I have pains and aches. My bowels do not move."

"Oh, well, you have constipation." That is the first thing that has been diagnosed. But do all these things exist without a cause? It would seem from one opinion that the "constipation" is the disease *per se,* but from another opinion it would appear to be the cause of disease; the "diagnosis" is made to apply to one as much as to the other. But this is the character of vagaries so common to Old School whims. These symptoms are but the language of nature, talking out as it were, and showing as clearly as the daylight the internal nature of the sick man or woman. If this state progresses the lungs break down. The doctor says, "Oh, now you have consumption;" or a great change appears in the liver, and he says, "Oh, now you have fatty degeneration of the liver;" or albumin appears in the urine, and he tells the patient, "Now I am able to name your disease. You have some one of the forms of Bright's disease." It is nonsense to say that prior to the localization of disease, the patient is not sick. Does is not seem clear that this patient has been sick, and very sick, even from childhood? Under traditional methods it is necessary that a diagnosis be made before the treatment can be settled, but in most cases the diagnosis cannot be made until the results of disease have rendered the patient incurable.

Again, take the nervous child. It has wild dreams, twitching, restless sleep, nervous excitement, hysterical manifestations, but if we examine all the organs of the body we will find nothing the matter with them. This sickness, however, which is present, if allowed to go on uncured, will in twenty or thirty years result in tissue change; the organs will become affected and then it will be said that the body is diseased; but the individual has been sick from the beginning. It is a question whether we will start out and consider the results of disease or begin at the beginning with the causes. If we have material ideas of disease we will have material ideas of the means of cure. If we believe an organ is sick and alone constitutes the disease, we must feel that if we could remove the organ we would cure the patient. A man has s necrotic condition of the hand; then if we believe that only the hand is sick we would think we had cured the patient by removing his hand. Say the hand is cancerous. According to this idea it is cancerous in itself and from itself, and seeing he would later die from the cancer of his hand we would conscientiously remove the hand and so cure the patient. For an eruption on the skin we would use local means to stimulate the functions of the skin and make it heal, and believing the eruption had no cause behind it we would conscientiously think we had cured the patient. But this is the *reductio ad absurdum,* for nothing exits without a cause. The organs are not the man. The man is prior to the organs. From first to last is the order of sickness as well as the order of cure. From man to his organs and not from organs to the man.

Well, then who is this sick man? The tissues could not become sick unless something prior to them had been deranged and so make them sick. What is there of this man that can be called the internal man? What is there that can be removed so that the whole that is physical may be left behind? We say that man dies but he leaves his body behind. We dissect the body and find all of his organs. Everything that we know by the senses belongs to physical man, everything that we can feel with the fingers and see with the eyes he leaves behind. The real sick man is prior to the sick body and we must conclude that the sick man be somewhere in that portion which is not left behind. That which is carried away is primary and that which is left behind is ultimate. We say the man feels, sees, tastes, hears, he thinks and he lives, but these are only outward manifestations of thinking and living. The man wills and understands; the cadaver does not will and does not understand; then that which takes its departure is that which knows and wills. It is *that* which can be changed and is prior to the body.

The combination of these two, the will and the understanding, constitute man; conjoined they make life and activity, they manufacture the body and cause all things of the body. With the will and understanding operating in order we have a healthy man. It is not our purpose to go behind the will and the understanding, to go prior to these. It is enough to say that they were created. Then man is the will and the understanding, and the house which he lives in is his body.

We must, to be scientific homoeopaths, recognize that the muscles, the nerves, the ligaments and the other parts of man's frame are a picture and manifest to the intelligent physician the internal man. Both the dead and the living body are to be considered, not from the body to the life, but from the life to the body. If you were to describe the difference between two human faces, their character and everything you observe of their action, you would be describing scarcely more than the will. The will is expressed in the face; its result is implanted on the countenance. Have you ever studied the face of an individual who has grown up a murderer or villain of some sort? Is there no difference between his face and that of one who has the will to do good, to live uprightly? Go down into the lowest parts of our great city and study the faces of these people. These people are night prowlers; they are up late at night studying villainy. If we inquire into it we will see that their affections are of that kind. They have the stamp upon their faces. They have evil affections and an evil face. The countenance then is expressive of the heart. Allopathic pathology recognizes nothing but man's body. Yet one can easily confuse the allopath by asking him what man's thought is, what man is. The homoeopath must master these things before he can perceive the nature of the cause of disease and before he can understand what cure is.

It is the sole duty of the physician to heal the sick. It is not his sole duty to heal the results of sickness, but the sickness itself. When the man himself has been restored to health. There will be restored harmony in the tissues and in the activities. Then the sole duty of the physician is to put in order the interior of the economy i.e., the will and understanding conjoined. Tissue changes are of the body and are the results of disease. They are not the disease. Hahnemann once said, "There are no diseases, but sick people," from which it is clear that Hahnemann understood that the diseases so-called, *e.g.*, Bright's disease, liver disease, etc, were but the grosser forms of disease results, viz., appearances of disease. There is first disorder of government, and this proceeds from within outward until we have pathological changes in the tissues. In the practice of medicine today the idea of government is not found, and the tissue changes only are taken into accounts.

He who considers disease results to be the disease itself, and expects to do away with these as disease, is insane. It is an insanity in medicine, an insanity that has grown out of the milder forms of mental disorder in science, crazy whims. The bacteria are results of disease. In the course of time we will be able to show perfectly that the microscopical little fellows are not the disease cause, but that they come after, that they are scavengers accompanying the disease, and that they are perfectly harmless in every respect. They are the outcome of the disease, are present wherever the disease is, and by the microscope it has been discovered that every pathological result has its corresponding bacteria. The Old School consider these the cause, but we will be able to show that disease cause is much more subtle than anything that can be shown by a microscope. We will be able to show you by a process of reasoning step by step, the folly of hunting for disease cause by the implements of the senses.

In a note Hahnemann says: "The physician's mission is not however, to construct so-called systems, by interweaving empty speculations and hypotheses concerning the internal essential nature of the vital processes and the mode in which diseases originate in the invisible interior of the organism," etc. We know that in the present day people are perfectly satisfied if they can find the name of the disease they are supposed to have, an idea cloaked in some wonderful technicality. An old Irishman walked into the clinic one day, and after giving his symptoms, said, "Doctor, what is the matter with me?" The physician answered, "Why, you have *Nux*

Vomica," that being his remedy. Whereupon the old man said, "Well, I did think I had some wonderful disease or other." That is an outgrowth of the old-fashioned folly of naming sickness. Except in a few acute diseases no diagnosis can be made and no diagnosis need be made except that the patient is sick. The more one thinks of the name of a disease so-called the more one is beclouded in the search for a remedy, for then the mind is only upon the result of the disease, and not upon the image expressed in symptoms.

A patient of twenty-five years of age, with gravest inheritances, with twenty pages of symptoms, and with only symptoms to furnish an image of sickness, is perfectly curable if treated in time. After being treated there will be no pathological results; he will go on to old age without any tissue destruction. But that patient if not cured at that early age will take on disease results in accordance with the circumstances of his life and his inheritances. If he is a chimney sweep he will be subject to the disease peculiar to chimney sweeps. If she is a housemaid she will be subject to the disease peculiar to housemaids, etc. That patient has the same disease he had when he was born. This array of symptoms represents the same state before the pathological conditions have been formed as after. And it is true, if he has liver disease or brain disease or any of the many tissue changes that they call disease, you must go back and procure these very symptoms before you can make a prescription. Prescribing for the results of disease causes changes in the results of disease, but not in the sickness except to hurry its progress.

We will see peculiarities running through families. In the beginning is the primary state which is presented only by signs and symptoms, and the whole family needs the same remedy or a cognate of that remedy; but in one member of the family the condition runs to cancer, in another to phthisis, etc., but all from the same common foundation. This fundamental condition which underlies the diseases of the human race must be understood. Without a knowledge of this it will be impossible to understand the acute miasmatic diseases, which will be considered later.

It is a well-known fact that some persons are susceptible to one thing and some to another. If an epidemic comes upon the land only a few come down with it. Why are some protected and why do others take it? These things must be settled by the doctrines of homoeopathy. Idiosyncrasies must be accounted for. Many physicians waste their time searching after the things that make their patients sick. The sick man will be made sick under every circumstance, whereas the healthy man could live in a lazaretto. It is not the principal business of the physician to be hunting in the rivers and the cellars and examining the food we eat for the cause of disease. It is his duty to hunt out the symptoms of sickness until a remedy is found that covers the disorder. That remedy, which will produce on healthy man similar symptoms, is the master of the situation, is the necessary antidote, will overcome the sickness, restore the will and understanding to order and cure the patient.

To get at the real nature of the human economy, and to lead up from that to sickness, opens out a field for investigation in a most scientific way. Sickness can be learned by the study of the provings of drugs upon the healthy economy. Hahnemann made use of the information thus obtained when he stated that the mind is the key to the man. The symptoms of the mind have been found by all his followers to be the most important symptoms in a remedy and in a sickness. Man consists in what he thinks and what he loves and there is nothing else in man. If these two grand parts of man, the will and understanding, be separated it means insanity, disorder, death. All medicines operate upon the will and understanding first (sometimes extensively on both) affecting man in his ability to think or to will, and ultimately upon the tissues, the functions and sensations. In the study of *Aurum* we find the *affections* are most disturbed by that drug. Man's highest possible love is for his life. *Aurum* so destroys this that he does not love his life, he will commit suicide. *Argentum* on the other hand so destroys man's *understanding* that he is no longer rational; his memory is entirely ruined. So with every proved drug in the Materia Medica, we see them affecting first man's mind, and proceeding from the mind to the physical economy, to the outermost, to the skin, the hair, the nails. If medicines are not thus studied you will have no knowledge of them that you can carry with you. The Materia Medica has been established upon this basis.

Sickness must therefore be examined by a thorough scrutiny of the elements that make up morbid changes that exist in the likeness of drug symptoms. To the extent that drugs in provings upon healthy men have brought out symptoms on animal ultimates must we study sickness with the hope of adjusting remedies to sickness in man under the law of similars. Ultimate symptoms, function symptoms, sensorium symptoms and mind symptoms are all useful and none should be overlooked. The idea of sickness in man must be formed from the idea of sickness perceived in our Materia Medica. As we perceive the nature of sickness in a drug image, so must be perceive the nature of the sickness in a human being to be healed.

Therefore our idea of pathology must be adjusted to such a Materia Medica as we possess, and it must be discovered wherein these are similar in order to heal the sick. The totality of the symptoms written out carefully is all that we know of the internal nature of sickness. Then the proper administration of the similar remedy will constitute the art of healing.

Classroom Notes

The sick

Everything that exists does so because of something prior to it.

Only in this way we can trace cause and effect, in a series of beginning to end and back again from end to the beginning.

What is meant by sick?

It is the man (individual) to be restored to health, not his body, not his tissues. If we have material ideas of diseases, we will have material ideas of the means of cure.

The organs do not make an individual. The individual is prior to his organs. From man to organs, is the order of sickness as well as the order of cure, and recovery ensues in this order only.

The will and understanding, constitute an individual.

That is the esse (internal) and exsisterae (external) constitute an individual. It is the non-material and material that makes an individual, which means that the substance and form constitute an individual.

Thus we can say that the soul (substance) and the body (form) constitute an individual.

It may be mentioned here that Kent was an avid Swedenborgian and his concept of the inner nature of man is derived from Sswedenborg's philosophy.

The making of an individual

The 'Esse' (interior non-material forces) and the 'Exsisterae' (external physical body) make an individual.

The interior of an individual is made up of the will, understanding and memory, which govern the physical body by a voluntary principle.

Will and understanding are organic forms arising from purest substances residing in every part of the brain. Man's mind is man himself. Man's mind that is the will and the understanding is his spirit and the spirit is the man. (*Swedenborg's divine Love and wisdom*).

Derivatives of Will and understanding

Will (Emotional part of the mind)	Understanding (The Intellectual part of the mind)
- Emotions - Desires - Pleasure - Enjoyment - Appetite	- Thought - Perception - Reflection - Recollection - Intention towards a things

*"Out of will and understanding arise the **voluntary principle** which governs the physical body through the central axis taking into account the sensory and the motor phenomenon."*

Sensory Phenomenon	Motor Phenomenon
- Touch - Taste - Smell - Hearing - Sight	- Consent - Conclusion - Intention - Determination - Action

"A Homeopath must master these things before he can perceive the nature of the cause of disease and before he can understand what cure is".

—James Tyler Kent

LECTURE II

§ 2. The Highest Ideal of a Cure

THE subject this morning relates to cure, to what the nature of a cure is. It is stated in the second paragraph of the *Organon* that

---

§ 2. The highest ideal of a cure is rapid, gentle
and permanent restoration of the health, or
removal and annihilation of the disease in its whole
extent, in the shortest, most reliable and most
harmless way, on easily comprehensible principles.

If you were to ask a physician, who had not been trained in homoeopathy, of what a cure consists, his mind would only revolve around the idea of the disappearance of the pathological state; if an eruption on the skin were the given instance, the disappearance of the eruption from the skin under his treatment would be called a cure; if haemorrhoids, the removal of these would be called a cure; if constipation, the opening of the bowels would be called a cure; if some affection of the knee joint, an amputation above the knee would be considered a cure; or if it were an acute disease and the patient did not die, it would be considered a cure of the disease. And that is really the idea of the patient as it is derived from the physician. The patient will often wonder at the great skill of the physician in removing an eruption from the skin, and will go back again when the graver manifestations, the tissue changes threatening death, have come on as a consequence, and will say to the doctor: "You so wonderfully cured me of my skin disease, why can not you cure of my liver trouble?" But this very scientific ignorant doctor has made a failure: he has driven what was upon the surface and harmless into the innermost precincts of the economy and the patient is going to die as a result of scientific ignorance.

There are three distinct points involved in this paragraph and these must be brought out. *Restoring health,* and not the removing of symptoms, is the first point. Restoring health has in view the establishment of order in a sick human being; removing symptoms has not in view a human being; removing the constipation, the haemorrhoids, the white swelling of the knee, the skin disease or any local manifestation or particular sign of disease, or even the removal of a group of symptoms, does not have in view the restoration to health of the whole economy of man. If the removal of symptoms is not followed by a restoration to health, it cannot be called a cure. We learned in our last study that "the sole duty of the physician is to heal the sick," and therefore it is not his duty merely to remove the symptoms, to change the aspect of the symptoms, the appearance of the disease image, imagining that he has thereby established order. What a simple-minded creature he must be! What a groveller in muck and mire he must be, when he can meditate upon doing such things, even a moment! How different his actions would be if he but considered that every violent change which he produces in the aspect of the disease aggravates the interior nature of the disease, aggravates the sickness of the man and brings about an increase of suffering within him. The *patient* should be able to realize by his feelings and continue to say, that *he* is being restored to health, whenever a symptom is removed. There should be a corresponding inward improvement whenever an outward symptom has been caused to disappear, and this will be true whenever disease has been displaced by order.

The perfection of a cure consists, then, first in restoring health, and this is to be done *promptly, mildly* and *permanently,* which is the second point. The cure must be quick or speedy, it must be gentle, and it must be continuous or permanent. Whenever an outward symptom has been caused to disappear by violence, as by cathartics to remove constipation, it cannot be called mild or permanent, even if it is prompt. Whenever violent drugs are resorted to there is nothing mild in the action or the reaction that must follow. At the time this second paragraph of the *Organon* was written physicking was not so mild as at the present day; blood-letting, sweating, etc., were in vogue at the time Hahnemann wrote these lines. Medicine has changed somewhat in its appearance; physicians are now using sugar-coated pills and contriving to make medicines appear tasteless or tasteful; they are using concentrated alkaloids. But none of these things have been done because of the discovery of any principle; blood-letting and sweating were not abandoned on account of principle, for the old men deprecate their disuse, and often say they hope the time will come when they can again go back to the lancet. But the drugs of today are ten times more powerful than those formerly used, because more concentrated. The cocaine, sulphonal and numerous other modern concentrated products of the manufacturing chemists are extremely dangerous and their real action and reaction unknown. The chemical discoveries of petroleum have opened a field of destruction to human intelligence, to the understanding and to the will, because these products are slowly and insidiously violent. When drugs were used that were instantly dangerous and violent the action was manifest, it showed upon the surface, and the common people saw it. But the patient of the present day goes through more dangerous drugging, because it destroys the mind. The apparent benefits produced by these drugs are never permanent. They may in some cases seem to be permanent, but then it is because upon the economy has been engrafted a new and most insidious disease, more subtle and more tenacious than the manifestation that was upon the externals and it is because of this tenacity that the original symptoms remain away. The disease in its nature, its *esse*, has not been changed; it is still there, causing the internal destruction of the man, but its manifestation has been changed, and there has been added to this natural disease a drug disease, more serious than the former.

The manner of cure can only be mild if it flows in the stream of natural direction, establishing order and thereby removing disease. The direction of old-fashioned medicine is like pulling a cat up a hill by the tail; whereas, the treatment that is mild, gentle and permanent flows with the stream, scarcely producing a ripple; it adjusts the internal disorder and the outermost of man returns to order. Everything becomes orderly from the interior. The curative medicine does not act violently upon the economy, but establishes its action in a mild manner; but while the action is mild and gentle very often that which follows, which is the reaction, is a turmoil, especially when the work of traditional medicine is being undone and former states are being re-established.

The third point is "upon *principles* that are at once plain and intelligible." This means law, it means fixed principles; it means a law as certain as that of gravitation; not guess work, empiricism, or roundabout methods, or a cut-and-dried use of drugs as laid down by the last manufacturer. Our principles have never changed they have always been the same and will remain the same. To become acquainted with these principles and doctrines, with fixed knowledges, with exactitude or method, to become acquainted with medicines that never change their properties, and to become acquainted with their action, is the all-important aim in homoeopathic study. When one has learned these principles, and continues to practice them, they grow brighter and stronger. The use of these fixed principles is the removal of disease, the restoration to health in a mild, prompt and permanent manner.

If one were to ask an allopathic graduate in this class how he could demonstrate that he had cured somebody, the answer could only be such as I have mentioned already, viz., that the patient did not die, or that the manifestations prescribed for had disappeared. If one were to ask a physician trained in homoeopathic principles the same question, one would find that there are means of distinctly demonstrating why he knows his patient is better. You would naturally expect, if it is the interior of man that is disordered in sickness, and not his tissues primarily, that the interior must first be turned into order and the exterior last. The first of man is his voluntary and the second of man is his understanding, the last of man is his outermost; from his centre to his circumference, to his organs, his skin, hair, nails, etc. this being true, the cure must proceed from centre to circumference. From centre to circumference is *from above downward,* from *within outwards,* from more important to less important organs, from the head to the hands and feet. Every homoeopathic practitioner who understands the art of healing, knows that symptoms which go off in these directions remain away permanently. Moreover, he knows that symptoms which *disappear in the reverse order of their coming* are removed permanently. It is thus he knows that the patient did not merely get well inspite of the treatment, but that he was cured by the action of the remedy. If a homoeopathic physician goes to the bedside of a patient and, upon observing the onset of the symptoms and the course of the disease, sees that the symptoms do not follow this order after his remedy, he knows that he has had but little to do with the course of things.

But if, one the contrary, he observes after the administration of his medicine that the symptoms take a reverse course, then he knows that his medicine has had to do with it, because if the disease were allowed to run its course such a result would not take place. The progression of chronic disease is from the surface to the centre. All chronic diseases have their first manifestations upon the surface, and from that to the innermost of man. Now in the proportion in which they are thrown back upon the surface it is to be seen that the patient is recovering. Here it is that the turmoil spoken of above follows the true homoeopathic remedy, and the ignorant to do not desire their old outward symptom to be brought back even when it is known as the only possible from of cure. Complaints of the heart and chest and head must in recovery be accompanied by manifestations upon the surface, in the extremities, upon the skin, nails and hair. Hence you will find that these parts become diseased when patients are getting well, the hair falls out or eruptions come upon the skin. In cases of rheumatism of the heart you find, if the patient is recovering. That his knees become rheumatic, and he may say : "Doctor, I could walk all over the house when you first came to me, but now I cannot walk, my joints are so swollen." If the doctor does not know that that means recovery he will make a prescription that will drive the rheumatism away from the feet and knees and it will go back to the heart and the patient will die; and it need hardly be stated that the traditional doctor does not know this, as he resorts to this plan as his regular and only plan of treatment, and in the most innocent way kills the patient. This is a simple illustration of how it is possible for the interiors of man to cease to be affected and the exteriors to become affected. If may be impossible for the man to be entirely cured, it may be impossible for this state to pass off, but that is the direction of its passing off and there is no other course. If the patient is incurable, while the means used are mild he may experience great suffering in the evolution of his disease, in the course of his partial recovery. To him it may not appear mild, but the means that were used were mild. In acute diseases we do not observe so much distress after prescribing as we see in old incurable cases, in deep-seated chronic complaints that have existed a long time. The return of the outward manifestations upon the extremities are noticed in such cases where they have been suppressed. To illustrate: there are many patients who have had rheumatism in the hands and feet, in the wrists and knees and elbows, who have been rubbed and stimulated with lotions and strong liniments, with chloroform, with evaporation lotions, with cooling applications, until the rheumatism of the extremities has disappeared to a great extent, but every physician knows that as the disappearance of his rheumatism progresses cardiac symptoms are likely to occur. When this patient is prescribed for, the rheumatism of the extremities must come back or the heart will not be relieved. That is true of every condition that has been upon the extremities and driven in by local treatment. Just as surely as you live and observe the action of homoepathic remedies upon man, so surely will you see these symptoms come back. The patient will return and say : "Doctor, I have the same symptoms that I had when I was treated by doctor so-and-so for rheumatism." This comes out in practice nearly every day.

It requires a little explanation to the patient, and if he is intelligent enough to understand it, he will wait for the remedy to act. But the physician who thinks most of his pocketbook will say: "If I don't give him a liniment to put on the limb he will go off and get another physician." Now let me tell you right here is the beginning of evil. You had better trust to the intelligence of humanity and trust that he will stay and be cured. If you have learned to prescribe for the patient even though he suffer, if you have learned what is right and do not do it, it is a violation of conscience.

This paragraph appeals to man's integrity; it is said in the last line "on principles that are at once plain and intelligible." Just as soon as you leave out integrity, and believe that a man can do just as he pleases, you leave out the foundation of success. But when these principles are carried out, when a man has made himself thoroughly conversant with the Materia Medica and thoroughly intelligent in its application, when he is circumspect in his very interior life as to the carrying out of these principles, then he will lead himself into a use that is most delightful, because by such means he may cause diseases to disappear, and may win the lasting friendship and respect of a class of people worth working for. He has more than that, he has a clear conscience with all that belongs to it; he is living a life of innocence. When he lives such a life he does not allow himself to wink at the notions that are carried out in families, as, for example, how to prevent the production of offspring, how to avoid bearing children, how to separate man and wife by teaching them the nasty little methods of avoiding the bringing forth of offspring. The meddling with these vices and the advocating of them will prevent the father and mother from being cured of their chronic diseases. Unless people lead an orderly life they will not be cured of their chronic diseases. It is your duty as physicians to inculcate such principles among them that they may live an orderly life. The physician who does not know what order is ought not to be trusted.

It is the duty of the physician, then, first to find out what is in man that is disorder, and then to restore him to health; and this return to health, which is a perfect cure, is to be accomplished by means that are mild, that are orderly, that flow gently like the life force itself, turning the internal of man into order, with fixed principles as his guide, and by the homoeopathic remedy.

Classroom Notes

The Highest Ideal of a Cure

1. **Restore Health:** When symptoms are removed there should be a corresponding inward improvement.

2. **Promptly, Mildly and Permanently:** The manner of cure can only be mild if it flows in the stream of natural direction establishing order and there by removing disease.

3. **Cure must be based on fixed principles:**
    That is, the cure should be:
    (a) From the center to circumstance,
    (b) From within outwards,
    (c) From above downwards,
    (d) From more important to less important organs,
    (e) In reverse order of appearance.

Unless people live an orderly life they will not be cured of their chronic disease. It is your duty as a physician to inculcate such principles among them that they may live an orderly life.

LECTURE III

§ 3. Perfection of what is Curable in Disease, Curative in Medicine and the Application of Last to First

---

§ 3. If the physician clearly perceives what is to be cured in diseases, that is to say, in every individual case of disease; if he clearly perceives what is curative in medicines, that is to say, in each individual medicine; and if he knows how to adapt, according to clearly-defined principles, what is curative in medicines to what he has discovered to be undoubtedly morbid in the patient, so that recovery must ensure-to adapt it as well in respect to the suitability of the medicine most appropriate according to its mode of action to the case before him, as also in respect to the exact mode of preparation and quantity of it required, and the proper period for repeating the dose; if, finally, he knows the obstacles to recovery in each case and is aware how to remove them so that the restoration may be permanent: *then he understands how to treat judiciously and rationally, and he is a true practitioner of the healing art.*

THE translator has correctly used here the word "perceive," which is to see into, not merely to look upon with the external eye, but to clearly understand, to apprehend with the mind and understanding. If Hahnemann had said "see" instead of "perceive," it might have been taken to mean seeing with the eye a tumor to be cut or, by opening the abdomen, to see the diseased kidney, or, by examination of the urine, to see that there is albumen or sugar present, by removing which in some mysterious way the patient would be cured. It is evident by this that Hahnemann did not look upon pathological change or morbid anatomy as that which in disease constitutes the curative indication. The physician must perceive in the disease that which is to be cured, and the curative indication in each particular case of disease is the *totality of the symptoms*, i.e., the disease is represented or expressed by the totality of the symptoms, and this totality (which is the speech of nature) is not itself the *esse* of the disease, it only represents the disorder in the internal economy. This totality, which is really external, a manifestation in the tissues, will arrange itself into form to present, as it were, to the physician the internal disorder.

The first thing to be considered in a case is, what are the curative indications in this case? What signs and symptoms call the physician's attention as curative signs and symptoms? This means not every manifestation is a curative indication. The results of disease occurring in the tissues, in chronic diseases, such as cancerous changes, tumors, etc., are of such a character that they cannot constitute curative signs; but those things which are curable, which are capable of change, which can be materially affected by the administration of remedies, the physician must know; they are the curative indications.

The physician ought to have a well-grounded idea of government and law to which there are no exceptions; he ought to see the cause of disease action to be from centre to circumference, from the innermost of the man to his outermost. If law and government are present, then law directs every act taking place in the human system. Every government is from the centre to the circumference. Look at it politically. Whenever the system of central political government is not bowed to, anarchy and loss of confidence prevail. There are also commercial centres. We must recognize

London, Paris, and New York as centres of commercial government in their different spheres. Even the spider entrenches himself in his web and governs his universe from the centre. There cannot be two governments; such would lead to confusion. There is but one unit in every standard. In man the centre of government is in the cerebrum and from it every nerve cell is governed. From it all actions take place for good or evil, for order or disorder; from it disease begins and from it begins the healing process. It is not from external things that man becomes sick, not from bacteria nor environment, but from causes in himself. If the homoeopath does not see this, he cannot have a true perception of disease. Disorder in the vital economy is the primary state of affairs, and this disorder manifests itself by signs and symptoms.

In perceiving what is to be cured in disease one must proceed from generals to particulars, study disease in its most general features, not as seen upon one particular individual, but upon the whole human race. We will endeavour to bring this idea before the mind by taking as an example one of the acute miasms, not for the purpose of diagnosis, as this is easy, but to arrange it for a therapeutic examination. Let us take an epidemic, say, of scarlet fever, or grippe, or measles, or cholera. If the epidemic is entirely different from anything that has hitherto appeared in the neighbourhood it is at first confusing. From the first few cases the physician has a very vague idea of this disease, for he sees only a fragment of it, and gets only a portion of its symptoms. But the epidemic spreads and many patients are visited, and twenty individuals have perhaps been closely observed. Now if the physician will write down all the symptoms that have been present in each case in a schematic form, arranging the mind symptoms of the different patients under "mind" and the head symptoms under "head," and so on, following Hahnemann's method, they - considered collectively - will present one image, as if one man had expressed all the symptoms, and in this way he will have that particular disease in schematic form. If he places opposite each symptom a number corresponding to the number of patients in which that symptom occurred, he will find out the essential features of the epidemic. For example, twenty patients had aching in the bones, and at once he sees that symptom is a part of this epidemic. All the patients had catarrhal affections of the eye, and a measly rash, and these also must be recorded as pathognomonic symptoms. And so by taking the entire scheme and studying it as a whole, as if one patient had experienced all the symptoms, he is able to perceive how this new disease, this contagious disease, affects the human race, and each particular patient, and he is able to predicate of it what is general and what is particular. Every new patient has a few new symptoms; he has put his own stamp on that disease. Those symptoms that run through all are the pathognomonic symptoms; those which are rare are the peculiarities of the different people. This totality represents to the human mind, as nearly as possible, the nature of this sickness, and it is this nature that the therapeutist must have in mind.

Now let him take the next step, which is to find in general the remedies that correspond to this epidemic. By the aid of a repertory he will write after each one of these symptoms all the remedies that have produced that symptom. Having in this way gone through the entire schema, he can then begin to eliminate for practical purposes, and he will see that six or seven remedies run through the picture, and, therefore, are related to the epidemic, corresponding to its whole nature. This may be called the group of epidemic remedies for that particular epidemic, and with these he will manage to cure nearly all his cases. The question now arises, which one is the remedy for each individual case? When he has worked out the half dozen remedies he can go through the Materia Medica and get their individual pictures so fixed in his head that he can use them successfully. Thus he proceeds from generals to particulars, and there is no other way to proceed in homoeopathy. He is called to a family with half a dozen patients in bed from this epidemic, and he finds a little difference in each case so that one remedy is indicated in one patient and another remedy in another patient. There is no such thing in homoeopathy as administering one of these remedies to all in the family because of a diagnostic name. Now, while one of the remedies in the epidemic group will most likely be indicated in many cases, yet if none of these should fit the patient, the physician must return to his original anamnesis to see which one of the other remedies is suitable. Very rarely will a patient demand a remedy not in the anamnesis. Every remedy has in itself a certain state of peculiarities that identifies it as an individual remedy, and the patient has also a certain state of peculiarities that identifies him as an individual patient, and so the remedy is fitted to the patient. No remedy must be given because it is in the list, for the list has only been made as a means of facilitating the study of that epidemic. Things can only be made easy by an immense amount of hard work, and if you do the drudgery in the beginning of an epidemic, the prescribing for your cases will be rapid, and you will find your remedies abort cases of sickness, make malignant cases simple, so simplify scarlet fever that classification would be impossible, stop the course of typhoids in a week, and cure remittent fevers in a day.

If the physician does not work this scheme out on paper he must do it in the mind, but if he becomes very busy and sees a large number of cases it will be too much to carry in the mind. You will be astonished to find that if you put an epidemic on paper you will forever be able to carry the knowledge of it in mind. I have done this, and have been surprised to find that after a dozen references to it I did not need it any more.

Now you may say, how is this in regard to typhoid fever? It is not a new disease, it is an old form. The old practitioner has unconsciously made an anamnesis of his typhoid cases, he has unconsciously written it out in his mind and carries it around. It is not difficult to work out the group of typhoid remedies, and from this group he works. The same is true with the regard to measles, certain remedies correspond to the nature of measles, i.e., when studied by its symptoms and not by name.

Of course, every now and then will come up a rare and singular case, which will compel you to go outside of the usual group. Never allow yourself to be so cramped that you cannot go outside of the medicines that you have settled upon as medicines, say, for measles. All your nondescript cases of course will get *Pulsatilla,* because it is so similar to the nature of measles, but it does not do to be too limited or routine, but be sure in administering a remedy that the indications are clear. Every busy practitioner thinks of *Ailanthus, Apis, Belladonna* and *Sulphur* for malignant cases of scarlet fever, and yet he has often to go outside of the group.

So the physician perceives in the disease what it is that constitutes the curative indication.

This presents itself to his mind only when he is clearly conversant with the nature of the sickness, as, for instance, with the nature of scarlet fever, of measles, of typhoid fever, - the zymosis, the blood changes, etc., so that when they arrive he is not surprised; when the typhoid state progresses he expects the tympanitic abdomen, the diarrhoea, the continued fever, the rash, the delirium and unconsciousness. These things stand out as the nature of typhoid. When, therefore, he goes to the Materia Medica he at once calls up before his mind this nature of typhoid, and so is able to pick out the remedies that have such a nature. He sees in *Phosphorus, Rhus, Bryonia, Baptisia, Arsenicum,* etc., low forms of fever, corresponding to the typhoid condition. But when the patient jumps away out of the ordinary group of remedies, then it is that he has to go outside of the beaten track and find another remedy that also corresponds to the nature of typhoid fever.

By these remarks I am endeavouring to hold up before you what the physician regards as the curative indications of disease. First he sees the disease in general as to its nature, and then when an individual has this disease this individual will present in his own peculiarities the peculiar features of that disease. The homoeopath is in the habit of studying the slightest shades of difference between patients, the little things that point to the remedy. If we looked upon disease only as the old-school physician sees it we would have no means of distinction, but it is because of the little peculiarities manifested by every individual patient, through his inner life, through everything he thinks, that the homoeopath is enabled to individualize.

"If the physician clearly perceives what is curative in medicines, that is to say, in each individual medicine." Here again he progresses from general to particulars. He cannot become acquainted clearly with the action of medicines individually until he becomes acquainted with the action of medicines collectively, proceeding from a collective study to a particular. This is to be done by studying provings. Suppose we were to start out in this class and make a proving of some unknown drug. It would be expected that you would all bring out the same symptoms, but the same general features would run through this class of provers; each individual would have his own peculiarities. No. 1 might bring out the symptoms of the mind more clearly than No. 2; No. 2 might bring out the symptoms of the bowels more clearly than No. 1; No. 3 might bring out heal symptoms very strongly, etc. Now if these were collected together as if one man had proved the medicine, we would then have an image of that medicine. If we had a hundred provers we would go through the whole nature of this remedy and perceive how it affected the human race, how it acted as a unit.

What I have said before about studying the nature of disease must be applied to the study of the nature of a remedy.

A remedy is in condition to be studied as a whole when it is on paper, the mind symptoms under one head, the symptoms of the scalp under another, and so on throughout the entire body in accordance with Hahnemann's schema. We may go on adding to it, developing it, noting which of the symptoms or groups of symptoms are the most prominent. A remedy is not fully proved until it has permeated and made sick all regions of the body. When it has done this it is ready for study and for use. Many of our provings are only fragments and are given in the books for what they are worth. Hahnemann followed up in full all the remedies that he handed down to us; in these the symptoms have been brought out upon the entire man. Each individual medicine must be studied in that way, as to how it changes the human race.

To understand the nature of the chronic miasms, psora, syphilis and sycosis, the homoeopath must proceed in identically the same way as with the acute. Hahnemann has put on paper an image of psora. For eleven years he collected the symptoms of those patients who were undoubtedly psoric and arranged them in schematic form until the nature of this great miasm became apparent. Following upon that he published antipsoric remedies which in their nature have a similarity to psora. To be a really successful physician the homoeopath must proceed along the same lines in regard to symphilis and sycosis.

Now, when the physician sees, as it were, in an image, the nature of disease, when he is acquainted with every disease to which we are subject, and when he sees the nature of the remedies in common use, just as clearly as he perceives disease, then on listening to the symptoms of a sick man he knows instantly the remedies that have produced upon healthy man symptoms similar to these.

This is what paragraph 3 teaches; it looks towards making the homoeopathic physician so intelligent that when he goes to the bedside of a patient he can clearly perceive the nature of disease and the nature of the remedy. It is a matter of perception; he sees with his understanding. When a physician understands the nature of disease and of remedies, then it is that he will be skilful.

Classroom Notes

What a Physician Must Perceive

1. The physicians must perceive that the causative indication in each particular case of disease is the totality of symptoms.
2. In such perception one must proceed from the generals to the particulars.
3. It is a matter of perception. A physician must see with his understanding.
4. When a physician understands the nature of disease and of remedies only then it can be said that he is skillful.

LECTURE IV

§ 4. "Fixed Principles." Law and Government from Centre

WE will take up today the study of the last part of the third paragraph relating to the *fixed principles* by which the physician must be guided. In time past, outside of the doctrinal statements of homoeopathy, medicine has never been matter of *experience*, and medicine today, outside of homoeopathy, is a "medicine of experience." Now, in order that the mind may be open to receive the doctrines, it is necessary that the exact and proper position of experience should be realized. If the true conception of law and doctrine, order and government, prevailed in man's mind he would not be forever hatching out theories, as they would not be necessary, and moreover he would be wise enough to know and see clearly what is truth and what is folly.

Experience has a place in science, but only a confirmatory place. It can only confirm that which has been discovered through principle or law guiding in the proper direction. Experience leads to no discoveries, but when man is fully indoctrinated in principle that which he observes by experience may confirm the things that are consistent with law. One who has no doctrines, no truth, no law, who does not rely upon law for everything, imagines he discovers by experience. Out of his experience he will undertake to invent, and his inventions run in every conceivable direction; hence we may see in this century a medical convention of a thousand physicians who rely entirely upon experience, at which one will arise and relate his experience, and another will arise and tell his experience, and the talkers of that convention continue to debate and no two talkers agree. When they have finished they compare their experiences, and that which they settle upon they call science, no matter how far they may be from the truth. Next year they come back and they have different ideas and have had different experiences, and they then vote out what they voted in before. This is the medicine of experience. They confirm nothing, but make from experience a series of inventions and theories. This is the wrong direction. The science of medicine must be built on a true foundation. To be sure, man must observe, but there is a difference between true observation in a science under law and principle and the experience of a man who has no law and no principle. Old-fashioned medicine denies principle and law, calls its system the medicine of experience, and hence its doctrines are kaleidoscopic, changing every year and never appearing twice alike.

Let me again impress the necessity of knowing something about the internal government of man in order to know how disease develops and travels. If we observe any government, the government of the universe, civil government, the government of commerce, physical government, we find that there is one centre that rules and controls and is supreme. A man has within him by endowment of the Divine a supreme centre of government which is in the grey matter of the cerebrum and in the highest portion of the grey matter. Everything in man, and everything that takes place in man, is prescribed over primarily by this centre, from centre to circumference. If man is injured from the *external, e.g.,* if he has his finger torn, it will soon be repaired; the order which is in the economy from centre to circumference will repair every wrong that is on the surface caused by external violence. The order of repair is the same in external as in internal violence. Injuries are external violence, but diseases are internal disorder performing violence. All true diseases of the economy flow from centre to circumference. All miasms are true diseases.

In the government of man there is a triad, a first, second and third, which gives direction, viz.: the cerebrum, cerebellum and spinal cord, or when taken more collectively or generally, the brain, spinal cord and the nerves. Considered more internally, we have the will and understanding forming a unit making the interior man; the vital force or viceregent of the soul (that is, the limbs or soul stuff, the formative substance) which is immaterial; and then the body which is material. Thus from the innermost, the will or voluntary principle, through the limbus of simple substance to the outermost, the actual or material substance of man, which is in every cell, we have this order of direction. Every cell in man has its representative of the innermost, the middle and the outermost; there is no cell in man that does not have its will and understanding, its soul stuff or limbus or simple substance, and its material substance.

Disease must flow in accordance with this order, because there is no inward flow. Man is protected against things flowing in from the outward toward the centre. All disease flows from the innermost to the outermost, and unless drug substances are prepared in a form to do this they can neither produce nor cure disease. There are miasms in the universe, acute and chronic. The chronic, which have no tendency toward recovery, are three, psora, syphilis and sycosis; we shall study these later. Outside of acute and chronic miasms there are only the results of disease to be considered. The miasms are contagious; they flow from the innermost to the outermost; and while they exist in organs yet they are imperceptible, for they cannot exist in man unless they exist in form subtle enough to operate upon the innermost of man's physical nature. The correspondence of this innermost cannot be discovered by man's eye, by his fingers, or by any of his senses, neither can any disease cause be found with the microscope. Disease can only be perceived by its results, and it flows from within out, from centre to circumference, from the seat of government to the outermost. Hence cure must be from within out.

In our civil government we see the likeness to this. Let any great disturbance come upon our government at Washington and see how, like lightning, this is felt to the circumference of the nation. How the whole country becomes shaken and disturbed as if by disease if it is an evil government. If the government be good, we observe it in the form of improvement, and everybody is benefited by it. If in the great centres of commerce, London, Paris or New York, some great crash or crises takes place, how the very circumference that depends upon these centres is shaken, as it were, by disease. Every little political office depends upon Washington, and that order must be preserved most thoroughly. The sheriff and constable, the judge and the court, are little governments dependent upon the law that is formed by the state. The law of the state would be nothing if the centre of our government at Washington were dethroned by another nation. All the law and principles in Pennsylvania depended upon the permanency and orderliness of the government in Washington, and there is a series from Washington to Harrisburg and from Harrisburg to Philadelphia. There can be no broken link.

It is now seen what is to be understood by order and directions, and that there are directions; nothing can flow in from the outermost to affect the innermost. Disturb one of the courts in Philadelphia and this does not disturb the country or the constitutional government. If the finger is burst this does not to any great extent disturb the constitutional government of the man, but the constitutional government repairs it. It is not a disease, it does not rack the whole frame. It is only that which shakes the whole economy, disturbs the government, which is a disease. So man may have his hand cut off without the system being disturbed, but let a little disease, measles for example, flow in from the centre and his whole economy is racked. Old-fashioned medicine talks of experience, but is entirely dependent on the eyes and finger; appearances are wonderfully deceptive. If you examine any acute miasm you may know what it looks like, but the *esse* of it cannot be discovered by any of the senses.

We have seen that everything is governed from the centre. Now what comes in the direction of law, what comes from principle, comes from the centre, is flowing in accordance with order and can be confirmed by experience. To apply it more practically, what we learn from the use of the law of homoeopathics, what we observe after learning that law and the doctrines that relate to it - all our subsequent experience, confirms the principles. For example, every experience with *Bryonia* makes *Bryonia* so much brighter in mind. With experience one grows stronger; one does not change or alter with every mood, but becomes firmly established. If every thing tends to disturb the mind, that means that you are in a state of folly or that you are insane; it may be a little of both. A man that relies on experience to guide him never knows; his mind is constantly changing, never settled; it has no validity. Validity is something absolutely essential to science. It is necessary for homoeopaths to look upon law as valid and not upon man, as there is no man valid. In homoeopathy it is the very principle itself that is valid, and things that are not in accordance with principle should not be admitted.

We see from all this the necessity of potentization. All causes are so refined in character, so subtle in their nature, that they can operate from centre to circumference, operate upon man's interiors and from the interior to the very exterior. The coarser things cannot permeate the skin. Man's skin is an envelope, protecting him against contagion from coarser materials; but against the immaterial substance he is protected only when in perfect health. In an unguarded moment he suffers, and this is the nature and quality of disease cause. It can only flow into man from the centre and towards the outermost in a way to disturb his government. The disturbance of government is a disturbance of order, and this is all there is of sickness, and we have only to follow this out to find that the very house man lives in, and his cells, are becoming deranged. Changes are the result of disorder and end in breaking down, degeneration, etc.; pus cells and the various forms of degeneration are only the result of disorder. So long as order and harmony go on perfectly, so long the tissues are in a state of health, the metamorphosis is healthy, the tissue change is normal, the physiological state is maintained.

We can only comprehend the nature of disease, and tissue changes the result of disease, by going back to its beginning. The study of etiology in the old school is a wonderful farce; because it begins with nothing. It is an assumption that tissue changes are the disease. From the doctrines of homoeopathy it will be seen that morbid anatomy, no matter where it occurs, must be considered to be the result of disease.

All curable diseases make themselves known to the physician by signs and symptoms. When the disease does not make itself known in signs and symptoms, and its progress is in the interior, we at once perceive that man is in a very precarious condition. Conditions of the body that are incurable are such very often as have no external signs or symptoms.

In the fourth paragraph Hahnemann says: "The physician is likewise a preserver of health if he knows the things that derange health and cause disease and how to remove them from persons in health." If the physician believes that causes are external, if he believes that the material changes in the body are the things that disturb health, are the fundamental cause of sickness, he will undertake to remove these, *e.g.,* he will cut off haemorrhoids or remove the tumor. But these are not objects Hahnemann means. The objects he means are invisible and can only be known by signs and symptoms. Of course, it is quite right for the physician to remove those things that are external to the sick man and are troubling him. These are not disease, but they are in a measure disturbing him and making him sick, aggravating his chronic miasm so that it will progress and destroy. These are outward obstacles and not the disease, but in this way man is very often rendered more susceptible to acute miasms. The things "which keep up disease" relate more particularly to external things. There are conditions in man's life which keep up or encourage man's disorder. The disorder is from the interior, but many of the disturbances that aggravate the disorders are external. The cause of disorder is internal, and is of such quality that it affects the government from the interior, while the coarser things are such as can disturb more especially the body, such as improperly selected food, living in damp houses, etc. it is hardly worth while to dwell upon these things, because any ordinary physician is sufficiently well versed in hygiene to remove from his patients the external obstacles.

In the fifth paragraph Hahnemann says: "Useful to the physician in assisting him to cure are the particulars of the most probable *exciting cause* of the acute disease, etc." The probable exciting cause is the inflowing of the cause as an invisible, immaterial substance, which, having fastened upon the interior, flows from the very centre to the outermost of the economy, creating additional disorder. These miasms all require a given time to operate before they can affect the external man, and this time is called the prodromal stage.

This is true of psora, syphilis and sycosis and of every acute contagious disease known to man. While the influx is upon the innermost of the physical man it is not apparent, but when it begins to operate upon his nerves and tissues, affecting him in his outermost, then it becomes apparent. Each miasm produces upon the human economy its own characteristics, just as every drug produces upon the human economy its own characteristics. Hahnemann says that these must be recognized, that the homoeopathic physician must be familiar enough with disease cause, with disease manifestations and drug manifestations to be able to remove them in accordance with principles fixed and certain. There should be no hypothesis nor opinion, neither should simple experience have a place.

If the physician is dealing with acute cases he must take into consideration the nature of the case as a malady, and so also with chronic cases. It is supposed that he is conversant with the disease from having observed the symptoms of a great many cases, and is therefore able to hold before the mind the image of the disease. When he is thoroughly conversant with the very image of the sicknesses that exist upon the human race he is then prepared to study Materia Medica. All the imitations of miasms are found in drugs. There is no miasm of the human race that does not have its imitation in drugs. The animal kingdom has in itself the image of sickness, and the vegetable and mineral kingdoms in like manner, and if man were perfectly conversant with the substances of these three kingdoms he could treat the whole human race.

By application the physician must fill his mind with images that correspond to the sicknesses of the human race. It is being conversant with symptomatology, with the symptom images of disease, that makes one a physician. The books of the present time are defective, in that they ignore symptomatology and do not furnish us an image of the sickness. They are extensively treatises on pathology, upon heredity, with very little of the patient himself. If we go back to earlier times, when the physician did not know so much about the microscope, when he did not examine into the cause of disease so minutely, we will find in such works as *"Watson's Practice"* much better descriptions of sickness. Watson stands at the bedside and relates what his patients look like, and hence it is a grand old book for the homoeopathic physician. Chambers, in his lectures at St. Mary's Hospital, London, also relates with accuracy the appearance of the patient. At the present time the old-school physician says: "I want to know nothing about your symptoms; take this and go to the first drug store and have it filled." This is the state of things at the present time, a look at the tongue, a feel of the pulse, and "take this," handing a prescription to be filled at the nearest pharmacy. Is that observing the sick? Can such a a man be the guardian of the sick, when it requires time to bring out every little detail of sickness, and a nervous girl is driven off and never permitted to tell her symptoms? Such patients have told me after an hour's conversation and taking of symptoms: "The other doctor told me I had hysteria, that there was nothing the matter with me, that I was just nervous." That is what modern pathology leads men to think and say. Everything is denied that cannot be discovered by the senses; hence this false science has crept upon us until it is a typical folly. As to the end of sickness, what sickness will do is of no great matter, because by the symptoms we have perceived the nature of the illness and may safely trust to the remedy. If no remedy be applied to check the progress of the disease it may localize in the heart, lungs or kidneys, but the *nature* of the sickness exists in that state of disordered government expressed by signs and symptoms.

Classroom Notes

Fixed Principles

Fixed principles with which a physician must be guided are:
1. Similia principle.
2. Cure can be comprehended by potencies.
3. All true diseases of the internal state flow from center to periphery. This is the order and direction of an individual.

Consciousness
The will and the understanding
(Interior of a person)
↓

Vital force
The Voluntary Principle
Immaterial formative life substance
↓

Material Body
(The exterior of a person)
The basic axis in the material body
The Cerebrum/ Cerebellum/ Spinal cord
↓

Connected via nerves and blood with
↓

Every cell of the body.

Man is protected against things flowing in from outward to the center. One example of each protective mechanism is the immune system.

4. All true diseases are miasmatic diseases.
5. The nature of sickness is such that it exists in disordered interior first and is expressed outwardly by signs symptoms.
6. Totality of symptoms is the only guide in order to perceive

what is to be cured in a disease.

7.   In perceiving what is to be cured, one must proceed from generals to the particulars.

8.   To understand what is curative in a remedy, it must be studied as a whole, as in provings and then only its principle or essence is truly understood.

9.   The physicians must know how to adapt the remedy to his sickness. To adapt the remedy a physician must:
     (a)   Match the totality of disease.
     (b)   Prepare the medicine in a right way.
     (c)   Dispense the medicine in right quantity (dose).
     (d)   Repeat the dose at the right time.
     (e)   Understand the obstacles to recovery and must remove them.

10. The cure should be in the following order:
     (a)   From center to circumference.
     (b)   From within outwards.
     (c)   From above downwards.
     (d)   From more important to less important organs.
     (e)   In reverse order of appearance.

Remember these are laws, the law directs and experience confirms.

"Experience has a place in science, but only a confirmatory place. It can only confirm that which has been discovered through principle and law guiding in proper direction."
To be sure a man must observe.

— **James Tyler Kent**

LECTURE V

§ 5. Discrimination as to Maintaining External Causes and Surgical Cases

WE wish to revert for a short time to the fourth paragraph, in which Hahnemann says: "The physician is likewise a preserver of health if he knows the things that derange health and cause disease, and how to remove them from persons in health."

The homoeopathic physician is a failure if he does not discriminate. It seems that among the earliest things he must learn is to "Render unto Caesar the things that are Caesar's" to keep everything in its place, to keep everything in order. This little paragraph might seem to relate to nothing but hygiene. One of the most superficial things in it is to say that persons about to be made sick from bad habits should break off their bad habits, they should move from damp houses, they should plug their sewers or have traps put in if they are being poisoned with sewer gas. It is everybody's duty to do these things, but especially the physician's, and we might almost let it go with the saying. To prevent coffee drinking, vinegar drinking, etc. is a superficial thing; but in this way he may preserve health.

To discriminate, then, is a most important thing. To illustrate it in a general way we might say that one who is suffering from conscience does not need a surgeon. You might say he needs a priest.

One who is sick in his vital force needs a physician. He who has a lacerated wound, or a broken bone, or deformities, has need of a surgeon. If his tooth must come out he must have a surgeon dentist. What would be thought of a man who, on being sent for a surgeon to set an injured man's bones should go for a carpenter to mend the roof of the man's house? If the man's house alone needs mending then he needs a carpenter and not a surgeon. The physician must discriminate between the man and the repair of his house. It is folly to give medicine for a lacerated wound, to attempt to close up a deep wound with a dose of remedy. Injuries from knives, hooks, etc., affect the house the man lives in and must be attended to by the surgeon. When the gross exterior conditions which are brought on from exterior causes complicated with the interior man then medicine is required. If the physician acts also as a surgeon he must know when he is to perform his functions as a surgeon, and when he must keep back as a surgeon. He should sew up a wound, but should not burn out an ulcer with Nitrate of Silver. If he is not able to discriminate, and on every ulcer he plasters his external applications, he is not a preserver of health. When signs and symptoms are present the physician is needed, because these come from the interior to the exterior. But if his condition is brought on only from external causes, the physician must delay action and let the surgeon do his work. Yet we see around us that physicians bombard the house the man lives in and have no idea of treating the man. They are no more than carpenters, they attempt to repair the roof, put on boards and bandages, and yet by their bandaging the man from head to foot they often do an improper thing.

The physician must know the things that derange health and remove them. If a fang of an old tooth causes headache day and night that cause must be removed. To prescribe when a splinter is pressing on a nerve and leave the splinter in would be foolishness and criminal negligence. The aim should be to discriminate and remove external causes and turn into order internal causes. A man comes for treatment, and he is living on deviled crabs and lobster salad and other trash too rich for the stomach of a dog. If we keep on giving Nux vomica to that man we are foolish. If a man who has been living viciously stops it he can be helped, but so long as that external cause is not removed the physician is not using discrimination. Vicious habits, bad living, living in damp houses are externals and must be removed. When a man avoids these externals, is cleanly, carefully chooses his food, has a comfortable home, and is still miserable, he must be treated from within.

You know how we are maligned and lied about. You have heard it said about some strict homoeopath, "He tried to set a broken leg with the c.m. potency of Mercury. What a poor fool!" But still outside of such an instance this discrimination is an important matter. You must remember it especially when busy, as at times it will be hard to decide. This kind of diagnosis is important, because it settles between things external and internal. Every physician does not discrimination thus, for if he did there would not be so many poultices and murderous external applications used. Among those who do not discriminate are those who apply medicines externally and give them internally.

Now we return to the fifth paragraph, which reads:

Useful to the physician in assisting him to cure are the particulars of the most probable *exciting cause* of the acute disease, as also the most significant points in the whole history of the chronic disease to enable him to discover its *fundamental cause*, which is generally due to a chronic miasm. In these investigations the ascertainable physical constitution of the patient (especially when the disease is chronic), his moral and intellectual character, his occupation, mode of living and habits, his social and domestic relations, his age, sexual functions, etc., are to be taken into consideration.

Little is known of the real exciting causes. Acute affections are divided into two classes (1) those that are miasmatic, which are true diseases, and (2) those that may be called mimicking sickness. The living in damp houses, grief, bad clothing, etc.; and the causes being latter have no definite cause, are produced by external causes such as removed the patient recovers. But the first, the acute miasms have a distinct course to run. They have a *prodromal* period, a period of *progress* and a period of decline, if not so severe as to cause the patient's death. Measles, scarlet fever, whooping cough, smallpox, etc., are examples of acute miasms. The physician must also be acquainted with the chronic miasms, psora, syphilis and sycosis, which we will study later. These have like the acute, a prodromal period and a period of progress, but unlike the acute, they have no period of decline. When the times and circumstances are favourable the chronic miasm becomes quiescent, but adverse times rouse it into activity, and each time it is aroused the condition is worse than it was at the previous exacerbation. In this paragraph Hahnemann teaches that the chronic miasms are the fundamental cause of the acute miasms, which is to say, if there were no chronic miasms there would be no acute. It is in the very nature of a chronic miasm to predispose man to acute diseases, and the acute diseases are as fuel added to an unquenchable fire. Acute diseases then exist from specific causes co-operating with susceptibility. We do not recognize measles or scarlet fever except in sick people. Their influence might exist in the atmosphere, but we cannot see it. So apart from the subjects that take and develop them we could not know that there were such diseases. If there were no children on the earth susceptible to measles we would have no measles, and if there were no chronic miasms there would be no susceptibility. We will take up the subject of susceptibility later.

Psora is the cause of all contagion. If man had not had psora he would not have had the other two chronic miasms, but psora, the oldest, became the basis of the others. The physicians of the present day do not comprehend Hahnemann's definition of psora, the think it meant an itch vesicle or some sort of tetter. They regard itch as only the result of the action of a bug that crawls in the skin making vesicles, all of which is external. This is quite in keeping with man's present form of investigation, because he can comprehend only that which he discovers by his senses. Hahnemann's idea of psora, as we shall see when we come to study it, is wholly different from these perverted views. Psora corresponds to that state of man in which he has so disordered his economy to the very uttermost that he has become susceptible to every surrounding influence. The other day I used the illustration of civil government, and said if our civil government is evil in its centre it will be in disorder in its uttermost. So if a man is evil in his very interiors, *i.e.,* in his will and understanding, and the result of this evil flows into his life, he is in a state of disorder. Let man exist for thousands of years thinking false theories and bringing them into his life, and his life will become one of disorder.

Later we will be able to show that this disordered condition of the economy is the underlying and fundamental state of the nature of psora which ultimates upon the body in tissue changes. Suppose a man starts out and believes that it is right for him to live upon a certain kind of food that is very distasteful to him; he lives upon that diet until he thinks (from his belief) that he really loves it, and in time his very outermost becomes as morbid as he is himself. When man is insane in his interior it is only a question of time and his body will take on the results of insanity because the interior of man forms the exterior. If the interior is insane the exterior is distorted, and is only suitable to the kind of insane or disordered life that dwells in it. False in the interior, false in the exterior so that the body becomes, as it were, false. This is speaking from analogy, but you will come to see that it is actually true.

Each and everything that appears before the eyes is but the representative of its cause, and there is no cause except in the interior. Cause does not flow from the outermost of man to the interior, because man is protected against such a state of affairs. Causes exist in such subtle form that they cannot be seen by the eye. There is no disease that exists of which the cause is known to man by the eye or by the microscope. Causes are infinitely too fine to be observed by any instrument of precision. They are so immaterial that they correspond to and operate upon the interior nature of man, and they are ultimated in the body in the form of tissue changes that are recognized by the eye. Such tissue changes must be understood as the results of disease only or the physician will never perceive what disease cause is, what disease is, what potentization is, or what the nature of life is. This is what Hahnemann meant when he speaks of the fundamental causes as existing in chronic miasms.

Just as soon as man lives a disorderly life he is susceptible to outside influences, and the more disorderly he lives the more susceptible he becomes to the atmosphere he lives in. When man thinks in a disorderly way he carries out his life in a disorderly way, and makes himself sick by disorderly habits of thinking and living. This deranged mental state Hahnemann most certainly recognizes, for he tells us everywhere in his teaching to pay most attention to the mental state. We must begin with such signs as represent to the mind the beginning of sickness, and this beginning will be found in the mental disorder as represented by signs and symptoms, and as it flows on we have the coarser manifestations of disease. The more that disease ultimates itself in the outward form the coarser it is and the less it points the physician to the remedy. The more mental it is the more signs there are to direct the physician to the remedy.

"In these investigations the ascertainable physical constitution of the patient, etc., are to be taken into consideration." This is the second state following the first one disordered. This deals with the outermost, it relates to externals. You have to consider both the internal and external man; that is, you have to consider causes that operate in this disordered innermost, and then the ultimates which constitute the outward appearance, particularly when the affection is chronic. These two things must be considered, the nature or *esse* of the disease and its appearance. At the present day diseases are named in the books from their appearance and not from any idea as to what the nature or *esse* of sickness is, hence the disease names in our books are misleading, as they do not have reference to the sick man but to ultimates. If the disease has terminated in the liver, numerous names are applied to the liver; if in the kidney or heart, these organs have names applied to them, and such terminations are called diseases. Consumption is a tubercular state of the lungs, which is but the result of an internal disorder which was operating in the interior long before the breakdown of tissue.

The physicians of these days will tell you that they go back to the cause, but they present no cause; they only bring up the superficial conditions that make the consumptive man worse. They will also tell you that a bacillus is the cause of tuberculosis. But if the man had not been susceptible to the bacillus he could not have been affected by it. As a matter of fact, the tubercules come first and the bacillus is secondary. It has never been found prior to the tubercule, but it follows that, and comes then as a scavenger. The cause of the tubercular deposit rests with the psora, the chronic miasm. Bacilli are not the cause of disease, they never come until after the disease.

Allopaths are really taking the sequence for the consequence, thus leading to a false theory, the bacteria theory. You may destroy the bacteria and yet not destroy the disease. The susceptibility remains the same, and only those that are susceptible will take the disease. Bacteria have a use, and there is nothing sent on earth to destroy man. The bacteria theory would make it appear that the all-wise Creator has sent these micro-organisms here to make man sick. We see from this paragraph that Hahnemann did not adopt any such theory as bacteriology.

This subject will be taken up in these lectures and fully illustrated, but I might throw out a few hints to set you thinking until we come to it again. We know that a dissecting wound is very serious if the body dissected is recently dead, and this we would suppose to be due to some bacteria of wonderful power capable of establishing such a dreadful erysipelatous poisoning that would go into man's blood and strike him down with a sort of septicaemia. In truth, soon after death we have a ptomaine poison, the dead body poison, which is alkaloidal in character, but we do not yet discover the presence of bacteria. The poison is there, and if a man pricks himself while dissecting that body and does not take care of the wound he may have a serious illness and die. But if after the cadaver has remained some time and become infected with bacteria, the dissector pricks himself the wound is not dangerous.

The more bacteria the less poison. A typhoid stool when it first passes from the bowel has a very scanty allowance of bacteria, and yet it is very poisonous. But let it remain until it becomes black with bacteria and it is comparatively benign. Why does the poison not increase with the bacteria? You can potentize, as I have done, a portion of a tuberculous mass alive with tubercular bacilli, and after potentizing it, after being triturated with sugar of milk and mashed to a pulp, it will continue to manifest its symptoms in the most potent form. You can precipitate the purulent tubercular fluid in alcohol, precipitate the entire animal life and potentize the supernatant fluid until you have reached the thirtieth potency, and having potentized or attenuated it until no microbe can be found, yet, if administered to healthy man, it will establish the nature of the disease in the economy, which is prior to phthisis. Thus we have the cause of phthisis, not in the bacteria, but in the virus, which the bacteria are sent to destroy. Man lives longer with the bacteria than he would without them. If we could succeed today in putting a fluid into the economy that would destroy the bacteria that consumptive would soon die.

The study of disease as to fundamental cause and apparent cause is an important subject. We cannot study cause unless we have first understood government associated with law. Hence recall to your mind that the *law directs and experience confirms.* Law is nothing but an orderly state of government from centre to circumference, a government in which there is a head. You show me a company that has no captain and you show me a disorderly company. Order exists from the highest to the lowest from centre to circumference.

Now I have led up to the point where you may ask, is it not disorder for man to settle what is true by the senses? Let us as homoeopaths turn our lives, our thinking abilities and our scientific life into order that we may begin to turn the human race into order. Let us adopt the plan of thinking of things from their beginning and following them in a series to their conclusions. No man is authority, but principle and law are authority. If this cannot be seen there is no use of proceeding any further with the study of homoeopathy. If man cannot see this he cannot see the necessity of harmony from centre to circumference, of government which has one head, and hence it would be useless for him to study the human body for the purpose of applying medicine to it. It must be accepted in this form or it will not satisfy man, it will not sustain his expectation, it will not do what he expects it to do; it will only accomplish what Allopathy has accomplished, viz., the establishment of confusion upon the economy.

Classroom Notes

Discrimination

Those Homeopathic physician are failure, who do not discriminate.

Remember:
1. One who has a sick conscience needs a priest.
2. One who has a sick vital force needs a physician.
3. One who has a deformity/ laceration/ broken bone needs a surgeon.

The Aim Should Be:
1. To discriminate and remove external causes.
2. To turn into order internal causes.

What are the causes of disease?

1. In acute disease: One must perceive what is the most probable *exciting* cause:
- Is it microbe?
- Is it environmental?
- Is it acute flare up of a latent miasm?
- Remember acute diseases exist from specific causes co-operating with susceptibility.

2. In chronic Disease: One must discover what is the *fundamental* cause, that is you have to consider both the internal and external of man. This is why you have to consider causes that operate in the disordered innermost, and the ultimates that constitute the outward appearance of expression of disease as signs and symptoms.

While studying the nature of chronic disease two things must be considered: nature of the disease (it's Esse) and appearance of the disease (it's Exsistre).

LECTURE VI

§ 6. The Unprejudiced Observer notes only change of State as shown by Symptoms

---

§ 6. The unprejudiced observer—well aware of the futility of transcendental speculations which can receive no confirmation from experience—be his powers of penetration ever so great, takes note of nothing in every individual disease, except the changes in the health of the body and of the mind which can be perceived externally by means of the senses; that is to say, he notices only the deviations from the former healthy state of the now diseased individual, which are felt by the patient himself, remarked by those around him and observed by the physician. All these perceptible signs represent the disease in its whole extent, that is, together they form the true and only conceivable portrait of the disease.

THE teaching of this paragraph is that the symptoms represent to the intelligent physician all there is to be known of the nature of a sickness, that these symptoms represent the state of disorder, that sickness is only a change of state and that all the physician has to do is correct the disordered state. Hahnemann, it seems, would say that it is great folly for a man to look into the organs themselves for the purpose of establishing a theory to find out whether the stomach makes the man sick, or whether the stomach makes the liver sick and such like. We can only end in theory as long as we think that way. So long as we set the mind to thinking about a man's organs and how these things are brought about we are in confusion, but not so when we meditate upon the symptoms of the sick man as fully representing the nature of the disease after these have been carefully written out.

Hahnemann starts out in this paragraph by speaking of "the unprejudiced observer." It would almost seem impossible to find at the present time one who could be thus described. All men are prejudiced. Man is fixed in his politics, fixed in his religion, fixed in his ideas of medicine, and because of his prejudice he cannot reason. You need only to talk to him a moment on these subjects and he will begin to tell you what he thinks; he will give his opinion, as if that had anything to do with it. Men of the present day cannot recognize law, and hence they are prejudiced; but when men have authority on which they can rest, then they can get rid of their prejudices. Suppose we have a large dictionary that we say is an authority on the spelling of words. If a club of one hundred and fifty men who bought that dictionary, and put it into a closet and say, "That is how we agree to spell," that is a recognition by these men that the book is authority. There would be henceforth no argument on the question of spelling. But if there were no authority one man would spell one way and another man in another way; there would be no standard of spelling. Such is the state of medicine at the present day, there is no standard authority. One book is authority in one school, and in another school they have another book, and so there is confusion.

Men cannot get rid of their prejudices until they settle upon and recognize authority. In homoeopathy the law and its principles must be accepted as authority. When we know these it is easy to accept them as authority, but seeing they are not known there is no authority and everybody is prejudiced. Men often ask, "Doctor, what are your theories as to homoeopathy? What are your theories of medicine?" I have no theories. It is a thing that is settled from doctrine and principle, and I know nothing of theory. A woman came into my office this morning and said, "Doctor, I have always been treated by the old school, but the doctors were unable to decide whether the liver made my stomach sick or the stomach made the liver sick." This is only confusion. No organ can make the body sick; man is prior to his organs; parts of the body can be removed and yet man will exist. There is no such thing as one organ making another sick. When we realize that the course of things is from centre to circumference we must admit that the stomach was caused to be in disorder from the centre, and that the liver was caused to be in disorder from the centre, but not that they made each other sick. One who has been taught such ideas cannot rid himself of them for a long time. It is a matter of years to get out of these whims and notions which we have imbibed from our inheritance. We cannot rid ourselves of confusion until we learn what confusion is.

In this paragraph Hahnemann does not speak of changes of tissue or changes in the organs, but changes of state. Man could see and feel tissue changes, but these do not represent to the intelligent physician the nature of disease or disease cause, they only indicate that because of the disorder within certain results have followed. The unprejudiced observer can see that pathology does not represent the nature of the disease, because numerous so-called diseases can present the same pathology and the same phenomena. The trouble is that there are so few unprejudiced observers. To get rid of our prejudices is one of the first things we must do in the study of homoeopathy. Therefore let me beg of you, while sitting in this room, to lay aside all that you have heretofore imagined or presumed, the whims and notions, and "what I thought about it," the things that you have learned from men and books, and only follow after law and principle, things that cannot deceive, cannot vary.

Even law will deceive if man is of prejudiced mind, because then he misreads the law and doctrine, and when things are called black they look to him white; every image is inverted in his prejudiced mind, because he realizes only with his senses, and sees with his eyes and feels with his fingers only the appearance of things, just as we say that the sun rises, judging from our eyes, although we know from our intelligence that it does not rise. If we believe our senses only we will accept all the notions of men. If the senses were invariable men would agree, but they are variable and no two men will agree in everything, for just as men's observations differ so different notions and theories will be established. We must try to get rid of the prejudices that we have been born with and educated into, so that we can examine the principles and doctrines of homoeopathy and seek to verify them. If you cannot put aside your prejudices the principles will be folly to you. The unprejudiced observer is the only true scientist.

"He perceives in each individual affection nothing but changes of state." The changes of state are such as are observed by the patient when he says he is forgetful, that his mind does not operate as it did, that he is often in a state of confusion, that when he attempts to deliver a sentence a part of it goes away from him, the idea passes away, or that he is becoming irritable, whereas he was pleasant, that he is becoming sad, whereas he was cheerful before, that there are changes in his affections, in his desires and aversions. These things relate to states: not to diseased tissues, but to a state of disorder or want of harmony. Dr. Fincke expresses it as "a distunement."

After the patient has related everything he can about his change of state, the physician may be aided by information from outsiders, from relatives who look upon the patient with goodwill, who wish him well. If the husband be sick it is well to get the wife's testimony. After the physician has written down all the information in accordance with the directions of § 85 for the taking of the case he then commences to observe as much as he can concerning the disorder, but more particularly those things which the patient would conceal, or cannot relate, or does not know.

Many patients do not know that they are awkward, that they do peculiar and strange things in the doctor's office - things that they would not do in health, and these are evidences of change of state.

The physician also notes what he sees, notes odors, the sounds of organs, chest sounds, intensity of fever, by his hand or by a thermometer, etc., and when he has gone over this entire image, including everything that can represent the disease, he has secured all that is of real value to him.

What if there are changes in tissue present? There is nothing in the nature of diseased tissue to point to a remedy; it is only a result of disease. Suppose there is an abdominal tumor, or a tumor of the mammary gland, there is nothing in the fact that it is a tumor or in the aspect of the tumor that would lead you to the nature of the change of state. The things that you can see, *i.e.,* the changes in the tissues, are of the least importance, but what you perceive in the patient himself, how he moves and acts, his functions and sensations, are manifestations of what is going on in the internal economy. A state of disorder represents its nature to man by signs and symptoms, and these are things to be prescribed upon.

Take a case which as yet has no pathological changes, no morbid anatomy, one that has only functional changes; the collection of signs and symptoms presents to the intelligent physician the nature of the state and he is clear as to the remedy. But if the patient does not receive that remedy, what will happen? The case will go on for a while, perhaps for two or three years, and when he returns to you on examination you will find that he has cavities in his lungs or an abscess in his liver, or albumin in the urine, etc. If it were the last, according to the old-fashioned notions and theories, you must now prescribe for Bright's disease; you would not think that remedy which you figured out two years before fitted his case perfectly then and is what he must have now. But he needed that remedy from his childhood, and you were able to figure it out from the symptoms of his change of state pure and simple, without tissue changes. Do you suppose because the disease has now progressed into tissue change, the organs are breaking down and the man is going to die, that this has changed that prim-

itive state? The man needs the same course of treatment that he
has needed from his babyhood. The same idea of his disease must
prevail now that prevailed before he had the tissue changes.
Bright's disease is not a disease, it is simply the ultimate or organic condition which has followed the progress of the original
change of state. Under other circumstances that change of state
might have affected his liver or his lungs.

Tissues changes do not indicate the remedy, and so as physicians we must learn to examine symptoms which are prior to morbid anatomy, to go back to the very beginning. Such a patient as I
have described must be looked upon as when he was in the simple change of state before matters were complicated. Besides this,
there is no manner of treatment for Bright's disease or any other
organic change. Our remedies appeal to man before his state has
changed into disease ultimates, and these remedies do not change
because morbid anatomy has come on, they apply as much after
tissue changes as before it. If we do not know what the beginnings
are we cannot in an intelligent way treat the endings.

In a footnote Hahnemann says, "I know not therefore how it
was possible for physicians at the sick-bed to allow themselves to
suppose that, without most carefully attending to the symptoms
and being guided by them in the treatment, they ought to seek and
could discover only the hidden and unknown interior what there
was to be cured in the disease, etc." The learned man in the old
school today would say, "Oh, I do not care anything about your
symptoms. I do not care if you are forgetful or irritable. If you do
not sleep I will give you something to make you sleep. But I must
sound your liver, for that is the cause of all your trouble, and I will
prescribe for that." He supposes the liver is the cause of all the
trouble, and believes that when that is corrected he has cured his
patient. What a false idea! His mind is upon mere theory. It is
common, when they do not know what has killed a man, to make
a post-mortem in order to discover the cause, and by this they find
out certain pathological conditions; but the aim of the physician is
to discover in his patient that just these conditions are present.

It is true, on the other hand, that the post-mortem affords the physician the means for a general study of the results of disease, which I would not, under any circumstances, prevent. Indeed, there are times when I would strongly encourage the study of morbid anatomy. The physician cannot know too much about the endings of disease; he should become thoroughly acquainted with the tissues in all conditions; but to study these with the idea that he is going thereby to cure sick folks, or that the things he picks up at such times are going to be applied in making prescriptions, is a great folly. It is astonishing that physicians should expect to find out by post-mortem and examinations of organs what to do for sick folks.

Physical diagnosis is very important in its own place. By means of physical diagnosis the physician may find out the changes in organs, how far the disease has progressed, and determine if the patient is incurable. It is necessary also in supplying information to Boards of Health. It may also decide whether you should give curative or palliative treatments. But the study of pathology is a separate and distinct thing from the study of Materia Medica.

In many instances foolish examinations are made. In the colleges women are examined with the speculum before a symptom is given, and if the mucous membrane is red the patient gets Hamamelis, and so on in a routine way through five or six remedies which cover all the complaints of women. Half a dozen remedies constitute the armamentarium of many of the eminent gynecologists. Such a practice as that does not cure, does not even benefit temporarily, it is simply an outrage. But bad though it is, perhaps it is not so great an outrage as is perpetrated when the physician imagines the disease is local, and that when he has cauterized it the woman is well, not realizing for one moment that these things come from a cause and that curing that cause should be his aim. Yet such is the teaching of the old school.

Now while the signs and symptoms are the only things that can tell the physician what the patient needs, and while those signs and symptoms relate to change of state and not to change of tissue, still there are signs that relate to tissue changes, and one who is acquainted with symptoms may consider these as indicating a change of state. For example, there are signs that indicate that pus is forming, there are appearances that will lead the experienced physician to know that the results of disease are coming; these are not valuable things in hunting for the remedy, but simply indicate certain conditions. The physician must learn to distinguish these from the symptoms that portray the state of the patient.

We are now prepared to see that if the patient is cured from cause to effect he must remain cured; that is, if the true inner disorder is turned into order he will remain cured, because this order, which is of the innermost, will cause to flow into order that which is the outermost and finally the function of the body to become orderly. The vital order will cause tissue order, because the vital order extends into the very outermost of the tissues, and tissue government and order is a vital order; so if the cure is from cause to effect, or from within out, the patient will remain cured. In incurable cases the effects may be removed temporarily or palliated, but the patient himself has not been cured as to the cause, and owing to the fact that the patient cannot be cured the old changes will return and grow stronger because it is in the nature of chronic cases to increase or progress.

Certain results of disease which remain after the patient is cured can be removed if necessary, but it is not well to remove them before the patient is cured. If a patient has a disease of the foot bones after a bad injury and the foot cannot be cured, first cure the patient, and then if the foot is so clumsy and useless that he would rather have a wooden one remove the foot. If you have to deal with a worthless honey-combed knee joint, joint, first cure the patient and then if the knee can never be useful and the limb is cold and the muscles are flabby consider the question of replacing it with an artificial one. If the economy after being turned into health cannot cure the knee nothing, that can be done to the knee, can cure it. Do not say that the patient is sick because he has a white swelling, but that the white swelling is there because the patient is sick.

Classroom Notes

The Unprejudiced Observer

The unprejudiced observer is the one who notes only change of state as shown by symptoms. In this paragraph Hahnemann does not speak of changes of tissues or changes in the organs, but changes of state.

How can we become unprejudiced observer?

1. After the physician has written down all the information (in accordance with paragraph 85) for taking the case then he must proceed to observe as much as he can, about the disorder, more particularly those things which the patient may conceal, or cannot relate, or does not know.

2. A physician must conduct full physical examination, which also indicates a change of state. A physician should be least bothered with tissue changes. There is nothing in the nature of diseased tissue to point to a remedy. It is only a result of disease.

3. Tissue change do not indicate the remedy, and so as physicians we must learn to examine symptoms which are prior to morbid pathology, and thus to go back to the very beginning.

If the internal state after being turned into health cannot cure the pathology nothing can be done to cure it.

LECTURE VII

§ 7. Footnote, Indispositions and the Removal of their Cause

IN a footnote to paragraph 7, Hahnemann writes:

> It is not necessary to say that every intelligent physician would first remove this exciting or maintaining cause (*Causa occasionalis*), where it exists; the indisposition thereupon generally ceases spontaneously.

You have, I believe, been led to conclude that there are apparent diseases, which are not diseases, but disturbed states that may be called *indispositions*. A psoric individual has his periods of indispositions from external causes, but these external causes do not inflict psora upon him. Such a patient may disorder his stomach from abusing it and thus create an indisposition. Indispositions from external causes mimic the miasms, *i.e.*, their group of symptoms is an imitation of a miasmatic manifestation, but the removal of the external cause is likely to restore the patient to health. Business failures, depressing tribulations, unrequited affection producing suffering in young girls, are apparent causes of disease, but in reality they are only exciting causes of indispositions. The active cause is within and the apparent cause of sickness is without. If man had no psora, no deep miasmatic influence within his economy, he would not become insane from business depression, and the young girl would not suffer so from love affairs. There would be an orderly state. The physician then must discriminate between the causes that are apparent or external, the grosser things, from the truer causes of disease, which are from centre to circumference. In every instance where Hahnemann speaks of true sickness, he speaks of it as a miasmatic disease, but here he employs another word. "Then the *indisposition* usually yields of itself," or if the psoric condition has been somewhat disturbed, order can be restored by a few doses of the homoeopathic remedy. To illustrate, if a man has disordered his stomach it will right itself on his ceasing to abuse it; but, if the trouble seems somewhat prolonged, a dose of medicine, like *Nux Vomica* or whatever remedy is indicated, will help the stomach to right itself, and so long as he lives in an orderly way he will cease to feel this indisposition.

"The physician will remove from the room strong smelling flowers which have a tendency to cause syncope and hysterical sufferings." There are some nervous girls who are so sensitive to flowers that they will faint from the odor. There are other individuals who are so psoric in their nature that they cannot live in the ordinary atmosphere; some must be sent to the mountains, some to warm lands, some to cold lands. This is removing the occasioning cause, the apparent aggravating cause of suffering. A consumptive in the advanced stages, one who is steadily running down in Philadelphia, must be sent to a climate where he can be made comfortable. The external or apparent cause, the disturbing cause in his sick state, is thus removed but the cause of his sickness is prior to this. The physician does not send the patient away for the purpose of curing him, but for the purpose of making him comfortable. "He will extract from the cornea the foreign body that excites inflammation of the eye, loosen the overtight bandage on a wounded limb that threatens to cause mortification, lay bare and put a ligature on the wounded artery that produces fainting, endeavour to promote the expulsion by vomiting of belladonna berries, etc., that may have been swallowed. Now, without the circumstances and surroundings in which Hahnemann stated these things, it has been asserted in the public prints that Hahnemann advised emetics. A class of so-called physicians have taken this note of Hahnemann's for a cloak as a means of covering up their scientific rascality, their use of external applications. They tell us Hahnemann said so, but we see it becomes a lie.

Here is another note: "In all times, the old school physicians, not knowing how else to give relief, have sought to combat and if possible to suppress by medicines, here and there a *single* symptom from among a number in diseases." This course of singling out a group of symptoms, and treating that group alone as the disease is incorrect, because it has no due relation to the entirety of the man. A group of symptoms may arise through the uterus and vagina, and one who is of this understanding has a plan for removing only the group of symptoms that belong to his specialty, whereby he thinks he has eradicated the trouble. Hahnemann condemns this doctrine, and we see at once its great folly. In many instances there are, at the same time manifestations of "heart disease," "liver disease," etc. (that is speaking in their terms; these are not diseases at all, as we know), so that every specialist might be consulted, and each one would direct the assault at his own particular region, and so the patient goes the rounds of all the specialists and the poor man dies. An old allopathic physician once made the remark about a case of pneumonia that he was treating, that he had broken up the pneumonia. "Yes," said another physician, "the pneumonia is cured, but the patient is going to die." That is the way when one of these groups of symptoms is removed; constipation may be removed by physic; liver symptoms may sometimes be removed temporarily by a big dose of calomel; ulcers can be so stimulated that they will heal up; but the patient is not cured. Hahnemann says it is strange that the physician cannot see that the removal of these symptoms is not followed by cure, that the patient is worse off for it.

Some patients are not sufficiently ill to see immediately the bad consequences of the closure of a fistulous opening but if a patient is threatened with phthisis, or is a weakly patient, the closure of that fistulous opening of the anus will throw him into a flame of excitement and will cause his death in a year or two. The more rugged ones will live a number of years before they break down, and they are held up as evidences of cure. Such treatment is not based upon principles, and close observation will convince a thoughtful man of its uselessness and danger. The fistulous opening came there because it was of use, and probably if it had been permitted to exist would have remained as a vent until the patient was cured. When the patient is cured the fistulous opening ceases to be of use, the necessity for it to remain open has ceased, and it heals up of itself.

The *Organon* condemns on principle the removal of external manifestations of disease by an external means whatever. A psoric case is one in which there is no external or traumatic cause. The patient perhaps has the habit of living as nearly an orderly life as it is possible for anyone to assume at the present day, going the regular rounds of service, using coffee and tea not at all or only in small quantity, careful in diet, removing all external things which are the causes of indispositions, and yet this patient remains sick. The signs and symptoms that are manifested are the true impression of nature, they constitute the outwardly reflected image of the inward nature of the sickness. "Now as in a disease from which no manifest exciting or maintaining cause has to be removed we can perceive nothing but the morbid symptoms, it must be the symptoms alone by which the disease demands and points to the remedy suited to relieve it."

Hahnemann's teaching is that there is a use in this symptom image, and every curable disease presents itself to the intelligent physician in the signs and symptoms that he can perceive. In viewing a long array of symptoms an image is presented to the mind of an internal disorder, and this is all that the intelligent physician can rely upon for the purpose of cure.

This divides homoeopathy into two parts, the science of homoeopathy and the art of homoeopathy. The science treats of the knowledges relating to the doctrines of cure, the knowledge of principle or order, which you may say is physiology; the knowledge of disorder in the human economy, which is pathology (that is, the science of disease, not morbid anatomy), and the knowledge of cure. The science of homoeopathy is first to be learned to prepare one for the application of that science, which is the art of homoeopathy. If we cast our eyes over those who have been taught, self-taught or otherwise, we see that some can learn the science, become quite famous and pass excellent examinations, and are utterly unable to apply the science, or, in other words, to practice the art of healing, for all healing consists in making application of the science.

We study disease as a disorder of the human economy in the symptoms of the disease itself. We also study disease from the symptoms of medicines that have caused disorder in the economy. Indeed, we can study the nature and quality of disease as much by studying the Materia Medica as by studying symptoms of disease, and when we cannot fill our time in studying symptoms from sick folks it is well to use the time in studying the symptomatology of the Materia Medica. True knowledge consists in becoming acquainted with and understanding the nature and quality of a remedy, its appearance, its image and its relation to man in his sickness; then by studying the nature of sickness in the human family to compare that sickness with symptoms of the Materia Medica. By this means we become acquainted with the law of cure and all that it leads to, and formulate doctrines by which the law may be applied and made use of, by arranging the truth in form to be perceived by the human mind.

This is but the science and we may, notwithstanding, fail to heal the sick. You will observe some, who know the science, go out and make improper application of the remedies, and seem to have no ability to perceive in a remedy that which is similar to a disease. I believe if they had a candid love for the work they would overcome this, but they think more of their pocket books. The physician who is the most successful is he who will first heal for the love of healing, who will practice first for the purpose of verifying his knowledge and performing his use for the love of it. I have never known such a one to fail. This love stimulates him to proceed and not to be discouraged with his first failures, and leads him to success, in simple things first and then in greater things. If he did not have an unusual affection for it he would not succeed in it. An artist once was asked how it was that he mixed his paints so wonderfully, and he replied, "With brains, sir." So one may have all the knowledge of homoeopathy that it is possible for a human being to have, and yet be a failure in applying that art in its beauty and loveliness. If he have no affection for it, it will be seen to be a mere matter of memory and superficial intelligence. As he learns to love it, and dwell upon it as the very life of him, then he understands it as art and can apply it in the highest degree. The continuous application of it will lead any physician or ordinary intelligence so far into the perception of his work that he will be able to perceive by the symptoms the whole state of the economy, and when reading provings to perceive the very nature of the sickness expressed in the provings. This degree of perception will enable him to see the "outwardly reflected image." You will not have to observe long, or be among physicians long, before you will find that many of them have a most external memory of the Materia Medica, that they have no idea of the nature of medicines they use, no perception of the quality or image of a remedy. It does not come up before their mind as an artist's picture; it is cold, it is far away. An artist works on a picture so that he sees it day and night, he figures it out from his very affections, he figures out every line that he is going to put in the next day, stands before it and he is delighted in it and loves it. So it is with the image of a remedy. That image comes out before the mind so that it is the outwardly reflected image of the inner nature, as if one man had proved it. If the symptoms do not take form the physician does not know his patient and does not know his remedy. This is not a thing that can open out to the mind instantly. You are, as it were, coming out of a world where the education consists in memorizing symptoms or memorizing key-notes or learning prescriptions, with really nothing in the mind, and the memory is only charged with a mass of information that has no application, and is only confusion leading man to worse confusion. There is no order in it. Hahnemann says: "In a word, the totality of the symptoms must be the principal, indeed the only thing the physician has to take note of in every case of disease, and to remove by means of his art, in order that it shall be cured and transformed into health." That is the turning of internal disorder into order manifested in the way we have heretofore explained, viz., from above downward, from within out and in the reverse order of the coming of the symptoms.

Classroom Notes

Indisposition

In every instance where Hahnemann speaks of true sickness, he speaks of it as a miasmatic disease. But here he uses another word "Then the indisposition usually yields of itself."

Causes of Indisposition

1. A Psoric miasmatic individual has his periods of indispositions form external causes, but these external causes do not inflict Psora upon him. For e.g.: Business failures, depressing tribulations, unrequited love, appear as causes of disease but in reality they are only exciting cause of indispositions. The active cause is within and the apparent cause of sickness is without.

2. If man had no deep miasmatic influence within his internal state, he would be able to throw off all these cares. He would not become insane with depression. There would be an orderly state.

Treatment of Indisposition

1. To correct this deep miasmatic influence on which *indispositions* rests, one requires few doses of Homeopathic remedy. The Organon condemns on the principle; removal of external manifestation of disease. Hahnemann's teaching is

that there is a use in this symptom image and in that image, every curable disease presents itself to the intelligent physician as signs and symptoms that he can perceive.

2.   In reviewing a long array of symptom an image is presented to the mind of an internal disorder and this is all that the intelligent physician can rely upon for the purpose of cure.

(a)   This divides Homeopathy in two parts:

• *The science of Homeopathy,* which treats the knowledge relating to the doctrine of cure, the knowledge of principle of orderly internal state (physiology), the knowledge of disorder in the internal state (pathophysiology) and the knowledge of cure.

• The science of Homeopathy is first to be learned to prepare one for the application of the science, which is the *Art of Homeopathy.*

As one learns to love the science and dwells upon it then he understands it as art and can apply it in the highest degree.

(b)   The continuous application of this art will lead any physician of ordinary intelligence so far into the perception of his work that he will be able to perceive by the symptoms the whole state of the internal disorder. While reading a proving he will perceive the very nature of the sickness expressed in proving. This degree of perception will enable him to see the *"Outwardly reflected image"* of the internal disorder.

If the symptoms do not take form in physician's eye, then he does not know his patient and does not know his remedy.

———————————

LECTURE VIII

§ 9. Simple Substance

---

§ 9. In the healthy condition of man, the spiritual
vital force, the dynamis that animates the material
body, rules with unbounded sway, and retains all
parts of the organism in admirable, harmonious,
vital operation, as regards both sensations and
functions, so that our indwelling, reason-gifted
mind can freely employ this living healthy instrument for the higher purposes of our existence.

THIS paragraph introduces the vital principle. It would hardly
seem possible that Hahnemann, in the time he lived, could say so
much in a few lines. In the seventh section of the first edition of
the *Organon*, Hahnemann wrote: "There must exist in the medicine a healing principle; the understanding has a presentiment of
it," but after the *Organon* had gone through a number of editions
Hahnemann had somewhat changed, and in this work, which is
the 1883 edition, he distinctly calls a unit of action in the whole

organism the vital force. You get the idea from some of his expressions that the harmony itself is a force, but I do not think that Hahnemann intends to teach that way. We cannot consider the vital principle as harmony, nor harmony as principle; principle is something that is prior to harmony. Harmony is the result of principle or law.

Hahnemann could perceive this immaterial vital principle. It was something he arrived at himself, from his own process of thinking. There was paucity of individual ideas at the time, i.e., ideas outside of the accepted sciences, but Hahnemann thought much, and by thinking he arrived at the idea contained in this paragraph, which only appears in the last edition, "In the healthy condition of man the *immaterial vital principle* animates the material body." If he had used the words "immaterial vital substance," it would have been even stronger, for you will see it to be true that it is a substance.

At the present day advanced thinkers are speaking of *the fourth state of matter* which is *immaterial substance*. We now say the solids, liquids and gases and the radiant form of matter. Substance in simple form is just as positively substance as matter in concrete form. The question then comes up for consideration and study: What is the vital force? What is its character, quality or *esse?* Is it true that man only has this vital force? Is it possessed by no animal, no mineral? For a number of years there has been a continuous discussion of force as force, or power to construct. The thought that force has nothing prior to it leads man's mind into insanity. If man can think of energy as something substantial he can better think of something substantial as having energy. When he thinks of something that has essence, has actual being, he must think of that *esse* as something existing and as having something which has ultimates. He must think in a series whereby cause enters into effect and furthermore into a series of effects. If he do not do this he destroys the very nature and idea of influx and continuance. If man does not know what is continuous, if he does not realize that there are beginnings, intermediates and ends, he cannot think, for the very foundation of thought is destroyed.

What do we mean by influx? As a broad and substantial illustration let us think of a chain. What is it that holds the last link of a chain to its investment or first attachment? At once we will say the intermediate link. What is it that connects that link? Its previous link, and so on to the first link and its attachment. Do we not thus see that there is one continuous dependence from the last to the first hook? Wherever that chain is separated it is as much separated as possible, and there is no longer influx from one link to the other. In the same way as soon as we commence to think of things disconnectedly we lose the power of communication between them. All things must be united or the series is broken and influx ceases.

Again, we see that man exists as to his body, but as yet we do not see all the finer purposes of his being.

To believe that man exists without a cause, to believe that his life force goes on for a while and does not exist from something prior to it, to think that there is not constantly and continuously that influx from cause whereby he continues to live, demonstrates that the man who does so is an irrational being. From his senses man has never been able to prove that anything can exist except it has continually flowing into it that which holds it in continuance. Then why should he, when he goes into the immaterial world, assume that energy is the first? We shall find by a continued examination of the question of simple substance that we have some reason for saying that energy is not energy *per se,* but that it is a powerful substance, and is endowed from intelligence that is of itself a substance.

The materialist to be consistent with his principles is obliged to deny the soul, and to deny a substantial God, because the energy which he dwells upon so much is nothing, and he must assume that God is nothing, and therefore there is none. But the one who is rational will be led to see that there is a supreme God, that He is substantial, that He is a substance. Everything proceeds from him and the whole series from the supreme to the most ultimate matter in this way is connected. Just as surely as there is a separation, and not a continuous influx from first to last, ultimates will cease to exist.

The true holding together of the material world is performed by the simple substance. There are two worlds that come apparently to the mind of man, the world of thought and the world of matter; the world of immaterial substance and the world of material substance. The world of material substance is in order and harmony. Everything that appears before the eye has beginnings. The forms are harmonious; every crystal of a metal crystallizes in accordance with order; man's very anatomy forms harmoniously. We see nothing in the material world to account for this, but we perceive that all things are held in position because of the continuous influx from first to last. There is no break in the chain and no break in the flow of power from first to last. Nothing can exist unless its cause be inflowing into it continuously. We see that all things made by man's hand decay and fall to pieces in time, but look at the things perpetuated from influx, look at their order and harmony from time to eternity, working by the same plan and in the same order.

There are many qualities predicated of simple substance, and one of the first propositions we have to consider is that simple substance is *endowed with formative intelligence, i.e.,* it intelligently operates and forms the economy of the whole animal, vegetable and mineral kingdoms. Everything with form goes on its natural course and assumes and continues its own private state. The laws of chemistry by analysis may be so revealed to man that he can detect all elements because they conduct themselves uniformly. The simple substance gives to everything its own type of life, gives it distinction, gives it identity whereby it differs from all other things. The crystal of the earth has its own association, its own identity; it is endowed with a simple substance that will establish its identity from everything in the animal kingdom, everything in the mineral kingdom. This is due to the formative intelligence of simple substance, which is continuous from its beginning to its end. If we examine the frost work upon the window we see its tendency to manifest formative intelligence. Plants grow in fixed forms. So it is with man from his beginning to his end; there is continuous influx into man from his cause. Hence man and all forms are subject to the laws of influx. If man is in the highest order and is rational, he wills to keep himself in continuous order, that his thoughts may continue rational; but he is so placed in freedom that he can also destroy his rationality.

This substance is *subject to changes;* in other words, it may be flowing in order or disorder, may be sick or normal; and the changes to a great extent may be observed or even created by man himself. Man may cause it to flow in disorder.

Any simple substance may *pervade the entire material substance without disturbing or replacing it.* Magnetism may occupy a substance and not displace any of it nor cause derangement of its particles or crystals. Cohesion is a simple substance; it is not the purpose of cohesion to disturb or displace the substance that it occupies. Therefore this first substance, or primitive substance, exists as such in all distinct forms of growths of concrete forms, and the material, concrete, individual entity is not disturbed or displaced by the simple substance; the simple substance is capable of occupying the material substance without accident to that substance or to itself.

When the simple substance is an active substance it *dominates and controls the body it occupies.* It is the cause of force. The body does not move, think or act unless it has its interior degrees of immaterial substance, which acts upon the economy continuously in the most beautiful manner, but as soon as the body is separated from its characterizing simple substance there is a cessation of influx. The energy derived from the simple substance keeps all things in order. By it are kept in order all functions, and the perpetuation of the forms and proportions of every animal, plant and mineral. All operation that is possible is due to the simple substance, and by it the very universe itself is kept in order. It not only operates every material substance, but it is the cause of co-operation of all things.

Examine the universe and behold the stars, the sun and the moon; they do not interfere with each other, they are kept in continuous order. Everything is in harmony and is kept so by the simple substance. We see co-operation in every degree, and this co-operation working in perfect harmony; we see human beings moving about; we see things going on about us on the earth; we see the trees of the forest making room for each other, existing in perfect harmony; the very sounds of the forest have harmony; and all this co-ordination is brought about by the simple substance. There is nothing more wonderful than the co-ordination of man's economy, his will and his understanding and his movements, which co-ordination is carried on by the life substance. Without this all matter is dead and cannot be used for the higher purposes of its existence. By the aid of simple substance the Divine Creator is able to use all created beings and forms for their highest purpose.

Matter is subject to reduction, and it can be continuously reduced until it is in the form of simple substance, *but it is not subject to restitution.* No substance can be returned to its ultimate form after it has been reduced to its primitive form. It is not in the power of man to change from first to last; that is, it is not in his power to ultimate the simple substance. This is retained for the Supreme Power Himself, from whom power continually flows through all the primitive substance to the end; *i.e.,* to ultimates. Now do you begin to see that the thing that does not start from its beginning with a purpose is not a thing, or, to put it another way, what makes anything a thing is because of its purpose or ultimate which is use, and there is never created a thing without a purpose. If it does not exist in continuous series from first to last it cannot be of use or of purpose; hence the end is in the first, and the end is in every succeeding link to its ultimate, the very form in which the use is to be appropriated and established. When you establish the first link in the chain you have the end of the next link in view.

The simple substances may exist as *simple, compound or complex,* and as such never disturb harmony, but always continue from first to last, and in that way all purposes are conserved. Throughout chemistry we can observe this compounding. We find Iodine uniting with its base; *i.e.,* two simple substances compounding in keeping, with their own individual plan, realiably and intelligently in accordance with the affinities for each other. When substances come together in that way they do not disturb the simple substance of each other, there is nothing destroyed, each one retains its own identity, and they can be reduced again to their simples by reaction and reagents. Now all of these enter into the human body and every element in the human body preserves its identity throughout and wherever found can be identified. Such combination, however, merely represents a composite state. But when these composite substances and simple substances are brought into an additional condition; *i.e.,* when they are presided over and dominated by something they may be said to enter into a very *complex* form, and in the body a life force keeps every other force in order. Dynamic simple substances often dominate each other in proportion to their purpose, one having a higher purpose than another. This vital force, which is a simple substance, is again dominated by another simple substance still higher, which is the soul. It has been the aim of a great many philosophers by study to arrive at some conclusion concerning the soul. They have attempted to locate it at some particular point, but we can see from the above that it is not in circumscribed location.

In considereing simple substance we cannot think of time, place or space, because we are not in the realm of mathematics nor the restricted measurements of the world of space and time, we are in the realm of simple substance. It is only finite to think of place and time. *Quantity* cannot be predicted of simple substance, *only quality in degrees of fitness.* We will see the importance of this in its special relation of Homoeopathy, by using an illustration. When you have administered *Sulphur* 55 m. in infrequent doses and find it will not work any longer you give the *c.m.* potency and see the curative action taken up at once. Do we not see by this that we have entered a new series of degrees and are dealing entirely with quality?

The sample substance also has *adaptation.* At this point man's reasoning comes up, leading to false conclusions from appearances, so that he has accepted what is called the environment theory. That the individual has an adaptation to his environment is not questioned, but what is it that adapts itself to environment? The dead body cannot. When we reason from within out we see that the simple substance adapts itself to its surroundings, and tends to adapt its house to the surroundings, and thus the human body is kept in a state of order, in the cold or in the heat, in the wet and damp, and under all circumstances. The surroundings themselves produce nothing, are not causes, they are only circumstances.

The life substance within the body is the vice-regent of the soul, and the soul in turn is also a simple substance. All that there is of the soul operates and exists within every part of the human body, and thus it is that simple substance acts as a vital force. The soul adapts the human body to all its purposes, the higher purposes of its being. The simple substance when it exists in the living human body keeps that body animated, keeps it moving, perfects its uses, superintends all parts and at the same time keeps the operation of mind and will in order. Let any disturbance occur in the vital substance and we see how suddenly inco-ordination will come. There is harmonious co-operation when the vital substance is continued in its normal quality; that is, in health what is more perfect than the human body in health, and what evidence have we of any greater wreck than the human body when it is not in health?

We see also that this vital substance when in a natural state, when in contact with the human body, is *constructive;* it keeps the body continuously constructed and reconstructed. But when the opposite is true, when the vital force from any cause withdraws from the body, we see that the forces that are in the body being turned loose are destructive. When these forces are not dominated and controlled by the vital force the body tends to decay at once. So we see that the vital force is constructive or formative, and in its absence there is death and destruction. If we examine the very simplest form of living organism, the plasson body, we will observe that it has the essentials of life, has everything in it that the very highest order of life has; it has the properties and qualities of the life substance of man and animals; it reproduces itself, it moves, it feeds, it is endowed with influx, and, lastly it can be killed. Now when you have said these things, you have predicated

much of the vital substance, or the highest and of the lowest. It
asserts its identity; it moves and feeds; it propagates and can be
killed. It does not sustain its identity by chemical analysis, because
when it is chemically analyzed it is no longer protoplasm.
Protoplasm is only protoplasm when it is living. Chemically, all
there is to be found of protoplasm is C.O.H.N. and S., but the life
substance cannot be found. You put together 54 parts of C., 21 of
O., 16 of N., 7 of H., and 2 of S., and what do you suppose you
will have? Simply a composite something, but not that complexity which we identify as protoplasm. In analyzing the protoplasm,
what has become of the life force? There is no difference in weight
after death; the simple substance cannot be weighed. Neither
weight, time nor space can be predicated of the simple substance;
and it is not subject to the physical laws, such as gravitation.

Now, when we consider this substance as an energy, a force, or
dynamis, - that is, something possessing power, - the subject is
intelligible. Inert elements have in their nature not only their own
identifying simple substance, but they have *degrees* of this identifying simple substance. The human body also has its degrees of
life substance, existing in degrees suitable for all its uses. The
innermost degrees of life substances are suitable to the will and
understanding, the outermost degrees to the very coarsest tissue,
and there is one continuous series of quality, in degrees from the
innermost to the outermost. Every cell has within it the innermost
and the outermost, because there is nothing in that which is coarsest but has that which is finest, too. The outermost envelopes are
dominated by the coarser degrees of simple substance, and the
innermost qualities are dominated by the innermost degrees. Each
portion has an appropriate form, and from the outermost to the
innermost it has all. Otherwise the human body could not be dominated or ruled by the soul. Each tissue has within it its portion of
the vital substance, each having its own peculiar kind of function.
Inert substances have their own degrees. *Silica* has its degrees of
simple substance within it, which can be brought out by the
process of potentization, whereby it may be continuously simplified, rendered finer and finer, so that each portion which remains

may, by continued potentization, be adapted to the higher degrees of the simple substance of man. The thirtieth potency of *Silica* will be sufficiently similar in form to reach in a curative way some of the diseases of man, viz., such as are dominating his economy in a correspondingly superficial and coarse series of the body. But it is true that *Silica* ceases after a time to act in the thirtieth potency, and it has to be further potentized in order that it may be similar in quality to the inner degrees, even until it reaches the very innermost or finest degrees of the simple substance.

Everything in the universe has its aura or atmosphere. Every star and planet has an atmosphere. The sun's atmosphere is its light and heat. Every human being has his atmosphere or aura; every animal has its atmosphere or aura. This aura is present in all entities. What may be said to be the aura of musk? That is a strong physical aura which almost everyone can perceive. A grain of musk has been kept for experiments' sake, in a bottle for seventeen years, giving off a perceptible aura yet without loss of weight. As a further evidence of aura, take, for instance, the animals which prey upon their food and you know that they can discover by an extremely intense aura states that man cannot discover. This is not an ordinary nose, but it is really the very instinct of the animal, whereby he perceives what is prey. His instinct is analogous to man's perception, any by this instinct he discovers his prey, when man would not be able to discover it. Man can discover musk in a bottle, but it is doubtful if man could discover the finest aura by its odor. This aura becomes useful and introduces a prominent sphere in the study of homoeopathics.

The consciousness between two simple substances is really that atmosphere by which one knows the other, and by which all affinities and repulsions between simple substances are known. They are in harmony or in antagonism. Human beings are thus classified by positives and negatives. Minerals and the world generally are classified by positives and negatives. This has an underlying cause. Substances are extremely powerful when meeting other substances that are antagonistic in any way, and also when meeting substances in a destructive way. The formative processes are often brought about by destruction; forms are destroyed in order that new forms may exist, and new forms therefore are often created from simple substance.

There are two realms or worlds, the realm or world of cause and the realm or world of ultimates. In this outermost or physical world we can see only with the eye, touch with the finger, smell with the nose, hear with the ear; such as the realm of results. The world of cause is invisible, is not discoverable by the five senses; it is the world of thought and discoverable only by the understanding. That which we see about us is only the world of ends, but the world of cause is invisible. It is possible that we may perceive the innermost, and it is important also that man may know and look from with upon all things in the physical world, instead of starting in the physical world and attempting to look upon things in the immaterial world. He will then account for law and perceive the operation of law. Homoeopathy exists as law; its causes are in the realm of causes. If it did not exist in the world of causes it could not exist in the world of ultimates. It is in the realm of cause that we must look for the primaries in the study of homoeopathy.

Of course it will be seen that the whole of this subject looks toward the establishment of a new system of pathology, which will be the groundwork of homoeopathy. All disease causes are in simple substance; there is no disease cause in concrete substance considered apart from simple substance. We therefore study simple substance, in order that we may arrive at the nature of sick-making substances. We also potentize our medicines in order to arrive at their simple substance; that is, at the *nature* and quality of the remedy itself. The remedy to be homoeopathic must be similar in quality and similar in *action* to disease cause.

Classroom Notes

On Simple Substance

(Simple substance or Immaterial formative substance).

In the healthy condition of man the Immaterial vital principle animates the material body.

Two Questions comes to the mind:

What is vital force?

What is its character, quality or esse?

The answer to theses questions can be perceived by thinking as follows:

1. If you think of energy as being substantial then think of something substantial as having energy.

2. If you think of something that has essence. Then why not think that esse is something existing and having ultimates.

3. You must think that everything is continuous, with beginning, intermediates and ends.

4. You must think in a series whereby causes enter into effects (that is to say series of effects). This is the nature and idea of influx and continuance.

5. All things must be united or a series is broken and influx ceases. (Remember lecture 1 states that every thing that exists does so because of something prior to it. Only in this way we can trace cause & effect.)

6. We shall see by a continued examination of the question of simple substance that we have some reason of saying that energy is not invisible per se but it is a powerful substance, and is endowed from an intelligence that is itself a substance.

7. If there is a separation, that is to say no continuous influx from first to the last, the ultimate will cease to exist.

8. The true holding together of the material world is performed by Simple Substance. There are two world that come to the mind.

The World of thought and the world of matter, the world of immaterial and the world of material substance, the world of causes and the world of ultimates.

The world of cause is invisible, only to be discovered by

understanding. It is the world of thought while the world of ultimate can be discovered by the five senses.

Homeopathy exists as law; its roots are in the world of causes. If it did not exist in the world of causes it could not exist in the world of ultimates.

It is in the world of causes that we must look for the primaries in study of Homeopathy.

Predicted Qualities of Simple Substances:

1. *Endowed with formative intelligence.*

   It intelligently operates and forms the internal state of the whole animal, vegetable and mineral kingdoms.

   Simple substances gives to everything its own type of life, gives them distinction, gives them identity whereby it differs from all other things. This is due to formative intelligence of simple substances.

2. *This substance is subject to changes.*

   That is, it may be in order or disordered. It may be normal or sick.

3. *Any simple substance may pervade the entire material substance without disturbing or replacing it.*

4. *When the simple substance is an active substance it dominates and controls the body, it occupies.*

   The energy derived from simple substance keeps every thing in order.

5. *Matter is subject to reduction.*

   It can be continuously reduced until it is in the form of simple substance.

6. *Simple substance may exist as simple, compound or complex.*

7. *Dynamic simple substances often dominate each other in proportion to their purpose.* One having the higher purpose than the other:

   Thus vital force, which is a simple substance and it is dominated by another simple substance still higher; which is the soul.

8.   *Simple substances are not subject to physical law* in considering simple substances we cannot think of time, place, space, weight or gravity.

9.   *Quantity cannot be predicted of simple substances, only quality in degrees of fineness can be predicted.*
     This has special significance in Homeopathic perception. Say after using 50M of Sulphur your response is leveled off and you now give Sulphur CM and curative action starts again. It is apparent we are dealing with quality here by entering a new series of degree (i.e. degree of fineness).

10. *Simple substance has adaptation.*
     Vital force adapts the body to its environment while the soul adapts the body to the higher purpose of its existence.

     (a) There is nothing more wonderful than the co-ordination of man's internal state, his will and his understanding and his movements. This co-ordination is carried on by the life substance, without which, all matter is dead and cannot be used for purpose of existence. The life substance within the body is the vice-reagent of the soul. The soul in turn is also a simple substance (the soul of man is in a spiritual body after it has cast off the material cover by which it was being carried out in this material world).

     (b) All that there is of the soul operates and exists within every part of the human body via simple life substance known as the Vital Force.

     (c) Now when we consider this substance as energy, a force or as something dynamic, that is something possessing power. We come to realize that inert elements have in their nature not only their own identifying simple substances, but they have degrees of this identifying simple substance.

     (d) The human body also has its degrees of life substance, existing in degrees suitable for all its uses.
          Every cell has within it innermost and outermost degree of life substance:

   (i) *Innermost:* The innermost degree of life sub-
      stance is dominated by finer degree of simple life
      substances, which are suitable to will and under-
      standing.

   (ii) *Outermost:* The outermost envelope is dominated
      by the coarrest degree of simple substances.

There is one continious series of quality, in degrees from the
innermost to outermost.

LECTURE IX

§ 10. and 11. Disorder First in Vital Force

§ 10. The material organism, without the vital force, is capable of no sensation, no function, no self-preservation; it derives all sensation and performs all the functions of life solely by means of the immaterial being (the vital force) which animates the material organism in health and in disease.

§ 11. When a person falls ill it is only this spiritual, self-acting (automatic) vital force, everywhere present in his organism, that is primarily deranged by the dynamic influence upon it of a morbific agent inimical to life; it is only the vital force, deranged to such an abnormal state, that can furnish the organism with its disagreeable sensations and incline it to the irregular processes which we call disease; for, as a power invisible in itself, and only cognizable by the effects on the organism, its morbid derangement only makes itself known by the manifestation of disease in the sensations and functions of those parts of the organism exposed to the senses of the observer and physician; that is, by *morbid symptoms*, and in no there way can it make itself known.

IT is clear that Hahnemann wishes to teach that it is a disorder of the activities of the internal man, a lack of harmony or lack of balance, which gives forth the signs and symptoms by which we recognize disease. These sensations constitute the language of disorder; *i.e.,* the means by which we recognize disorder and disease. This immaterial vital principle, this simple substance, everywhere pervades the organism, and in disease this disorder everywhere pervades the organism, it pervades every cell and every portion of the human economy. We will see in course of time that the change in form of a cell is the result first of disorder, that the derangement of the immaterial vital principle is the very beginning of the disorder, and that with this beginning there are changes in sensation by which man may know this beginning, which occurs long before there is any visible change in the material substance of the body.

The patient himself can feel by his sensations the changes, and this is inimical to life, and death immediately follows, for life in its fullest sense is freedom. As soon as the internal economy is deprived in any manner of its freedom, death is threatening; where freedom is lost death is sure to follow.

So it is when there is the inflowing of a simple substance that has the form or essence of a disease. It is in its essence an evil that is flowing in to the economy, but it is a simple substance. Everything is substantial or real, and has in itself operating and perpetuating power. The fact that it can operate and perpetuate is the evidence of power, and if it has power it results in something. Every cause of disease then has form. If it were not in the form of single substance it could not affect the forms of simple substance in the natural state of the economy. Moreover, it has its association, from the finest forms of physical substance to the crudest, from the finest forms of physical substance to the crudest, from beginning to end, from the inner to the outer. Such changes and activities as result in the very crudest forms are but the results of disease through a series of degrees, coarser and coarser to the outermost man. Everything that can be seen, that can be observed with the aid of the finest instrument, is but the result. Nothing in the world of immaterial substance can be seen with any faculty that is capable of seeing things in the world of material substance. The employment of instruments of precision will enable us to see the finest disease results, which are the outcome or results of things immaterial, the bacteria for instance, the very finest form of animal or vegetable life; but the cause of disease is a million times more subtle than these and cannot be seen by the human eye. The finest visible objects are but results of things still finer, so that the cause rests within. The morbific agents that Hahnemann refers to are simply the extremely fine forms of simple substance, or to bring them down to human thought we might call them viruses; but viruses are often gross because they can sometimes be observed by the vision of man, and therefore we must remember that within the virus is its innermost and that this innermost is in itself capable of giving form to the outermost, which is the visible virus aggregated and concentrated.

The coarser forms would be comparatively harmless were it not for their interiors. Disease products are comparatively harmless were it not for the fact that they contain an innermost and it is the innermost itself that is causative. The bacteria are the result of conditions within, they are, as it were, evolved by a spontaneous generation - literally, that is what it is. Every virus is capable of assuming forms and shapes in ultimates. The causes of ultimates are not from without but the immaterial invisible center. Those things that appear to man's eye are evolved, just as man himself is formed from a center which has the power of evolving, an endowment from the Creator, operating under fixed general laws. It is only when the vital principle is disturbed by cause of a disease character (that is the innermost of a virus in the form of a simple substance) that it gives forth any consciousness of itself.

If there were no disturbing influence in the interiors of man he never would have symptoms. As you sit there in your seats in a perfect state of quietude or tranquility you are not conscious of your eyes, of your limbs, of your hair. You have to stop and think whether you feel or not. When all the functions are carried on in a perfectly orderly way you have no consciousness of your body, which means that you are in freedom. When not in freedom the individual says. "I feel." It is this disturbance of an invisible character which comes from cause, and appears by changes in the activities of the body, changes in sensations, changes in functions. It is in accordance with all-wise Providence that these sensations should appear to the physician who shall be intelligent enough to read them and know what they mean. They are a warning, they are for us, for purpose. No feeling a man can have is without purpose, as there is nothing in the universe without its use. Hence these morbid sensations reveal to the physician that there is disorder.

To establish freedom should be the aim of the physician, and if a physician's work does not result in placing his patient in freedom he cannot heal the sick, for healing the sick is placing the patient in freedom, giving him absolute physical freedom. If the physician causes the pains to cease by a dose of Morphine, can we call that freedom? Is the patient not made stupid beyond the recognition of the nature of his feelings? The large doses of the old school produce anything but freedom. We must look elsewhere to find that kind of healing which turns disorder into order and makes man free. By removing the signs and symptoms in an orderly way, by converting disorder into order so that the symptoms no longer have a cause (for as we have already seen when the economy is turned into order it ceases to give forth symptoms), we place our patients in freedom, both physical and mental.

"Only the vital principle thus disturbed can give to the organism its abnormal sensations and incline it to the irregular actions we call disease." This is totally different from calling the results of disease the disease, e.g., calling Bright's disease, cancer, or palsy, diseases. Most of the conditions of the human economy that are called diseases in the books are not diseases, but the results of disease. To call a group of symptoms a disease of one part, and another group of symptoms a disease of another part, is a great heresy and leads to errors in prescribing that can never be corrected. Organic change is the result of disease.

Morbid disturbances can be perceived solely by means of the expression of disease in the sensations and actions! We would have no means of perceiving the morbid disturbance of the invis-

ible principle except by morbid sensations, and if these were not
present we would have no means of putting the patient in freedom. There are patients so sick that they cannot be put in freedom,
those for whom there are no means of cure, and in these, while the
internal structural changes are going on slowly, the morbid symptoms are not present. Such patients continually change doctors
and change climates, recognizing, as it were, that no one is capable of relieving them. With an incurable change in a vital organ,
all or most of the symptoms that existed go away; the symptoms
of the disease are suppressed, as it were, by the tremendous strain
upon the system.

This is particularly true of the malignant forms of disease
results. The symptoms that existed years ago have disappeared
and the patient says "Oh, they did not amount to anything; I had
had them all my life." But those are the symptoms that would
manifest to the physician the nature of the remedy, for they give
to him the real image of the sickness.

Some doctors say: "Oh, we will have a remedy for cancer some
day," having in mind only the symptoms of cancer; that is, the
symptoms that represent the results of disease and not the symptoms that represent the disease itself. There is a vast difference
between these two. These physicians would not talk so if they
only think in this proper and wholesome fashion, that to cure the
patient would be to cure and cancer, and in order to cure the
patient it is necessary to go back in his history and get those
symptoms that represent the patient in a state of disease and not
the tissues in a state of disease results. In the latter state, the original symptoms of the disease have often disappeared; they are as
it were, swallowed up. So it is when the innermost disease has
acted and the whole body is full of disease results, such as dropsical conditions, or pus sacs, or hip-joint abscesses. The pains
make the patient unable to think of his symptoms. Then these
physicians come along and prescribe for the resultant states and
end in failure. They give *Silica* for hip-joint disease and Bufo for
epilepsy, and so on, giving medicines for groups of symptoms.

That is not homoeopathy. Such men then go off and say: "Oh,

I have tried everything," but they have tried nothing but modern practice. It is a travesty upon homoeopathy. The expert physician can listen to signs and symptoms before morbid changes have taken place, and if no medicines have every been administered, if no drugging has been resorted to, no morphine and no other violent and vicious drugs, the image stands out before him in relief; it is perfect, because it has not been meddled with. It speaks with clearness, and the physician who is intelligent can learn to read it. But the physician who is not capable of seeing that this is different from the group of pathological symptoms that represent the so-called fixed diseases, if he cannot make a distinction between the symptoms that represent the disease *per se* and the symptoms that represent the result of disease, he will never practice homoeopathy successfully. If he cannot understand it he had better work at it until he does understand it; he must continue to labour until he can discriminate between the organic symptoms associated with the results of disease and the pure signs given forth by nature. Every few days I run across a homoeopathic physician who asks: "What remedy are you using in such and such case?" Such a thing has no place in my mind, and I look upon one who speaks in that way as a man untrained in homoeopathics. I truly have lost my patience over such things, for the old gray-heads, who have practiced for years and pretended to practice homoeopathy, do not hesitate to say that "the best remedy for epilepsy" is so and so.

What nonsense! That is not adjusting the remedy to the state of the patient that existed before he had these structural changes and fixed groups of symptoms, for if you adjust a remedy to the pathological condition you are not adjusting it to the patient, to his very beginnings down to the present time. He need not have pathological results, all he needs to have is symptoms. The patient can cure his own morbid anatomy. If you will take away the first state of disorder his economy will be safe. If the results of disease cannot be removed the patient himself will return to health and the morbid anatomy will undergo such changes that it will not affect his state of health. The fibrinous adhesions needs not necessarily go away a state of quiescence comes and remains year after year so long as he remains well.

To think of remedies for cancer is confusion, but to think of remedies for the patient who appears to have cancer is orderly, and you will be astonished to know what wonderful changes will take place in these conditions when remedies that correspond to the conditions before the cancer began are administered. Cancer is the result of disorder, which disorder must be turned in order and must be healed. We dwell upon this, for many paragraphs bring out this distinction between symptoms and results of disease. The true morbid sensations of a healthy organism are what we must first consider. It is first assumed that the organism is in a state of health and capable of performing its functions, and then the morbid sensations of this healthy organism are the symptoms that come to the physician as a forerunner of death in parts, and finally death of the whole. The patient tells the physician his sensations, of the numbness of his fingers, of the pricking in his skin, of the pain in his stomach, etc., all the sensations of any part of which he is reminded. The healthy man is not reminded of his parts. He passes his stool without pain in the part. If he has pain or bleeding he is reminded of this part. If he passes his urine without sensation we say it is normal and he is in freedom, but if burning and smarting and tenesmus follow he is reminded of it, and these sensations constitute symptoms.

If the patient is waxy and pallid, has papules and pustules, or swollen and varicose veins with red face, red eyes, etc., these the physician can see and note down. Again there are things that the physician cannot see and that the patient cannot tell, that the mother, sister, husband or wife should relate to the physician at his office. These symptoms constitute what there is knowable of the sickness, that which appears to the mind of the physician upon which he makes up his verdict. When the strong symptoms are all gathered together the physician in studying the case must separate out those things that were observed years ago from those things that are observed today, noting how they have changed and why changed. Sometimes they have been changed by drugs so that the whole nature of the economy is giving out a different group of symptoms.

The physician must learn the changes all along the line, from beginning to end; what symptoms represented this sick man ten years ago, and what symptoms represent him now. Perhaps now he has morbid anatomy, pathological conditions in his lungs, liver and kidneys. The physician who has been for twenty year observing previous and present conditions in this manner, by hearing the symptoms can practically locate the morbid anatomy; he can tell where it will appear, knows when pus is in organs and where, and he can for tell pretty well what is soon to go on in the economy. I would rather trust to a careful study of the symptoms than most physician's written diagnosis of phthisis, or organic diseases of the liver or of the heart. The symptoms do not lie, they do not exist from opinions of men who have thumped and pounded over the human body to find out what is going on inside, which is in many instances confusing even to the best diagnosticians. A considerable observation amongst medical men will lead one to discover that the dollar is the chief end of the practice of medicine when practiced in the old way; there is nothing else in it, nothing to admire or cherish.

To become conversant with symptoms, to judge of the sphere and progress of disease by the study of symptomatology, is the requirement necessary for the homoeopath. Of course, bystanders will say to the patient, "That doctor cannot know much; he did not give you a physical examination." After the examination of the symptoms has been made there is no reason why you should not make a physical examination of the patient; but do not let this deprive you of becoming thoroughly educated in studying symptoms, because the real study of sickness is the meditation of his symptoms, and to become wise in symptoms is to become an able prescriber. Study physical diagnosis to your heart's content, but weigh carefully what you discover and compare it with the symptoms in order to ascertain what the different symptoms mean. You cannot study the symptoms of man without becoming extremely well acquainted with the nervous system. The anatomy of the nerves and of the brain should be thoroughly known. Not always that you may name the nerve, but that you may know where it is and what its functions are, and this study should be continued throughout all your life. The physician should be conversant with anatomy and physiology, but by studying the symptomatology he acquires a knowledge of physiology which it is impossible to obtain in any other way; he acquires a knowledge of the functions and operations of arteries, nerves and muscles because they call attention to themselves when in disturbance, and he sees therefore how the symptoms manifest themselves. By studying the symptom in the recorded pathogenesis one may learn much about true pathology. Morbid anatomy furnishes no basis for prescribing, but true pathology is often of the greatest benefit, helping the image of the sickness to shape itself before the mind.

Classroom Notes

Disorder First in Vital Force

Hahnemann wishes to teach us that it is disorder of the activities of the internal man, a lack of harmony or a lack of balance, which gives forth the sign and symptoms, by which we recognize disease.

These sensations constitute the language of disorder. That is the language of signs & symptoms should be the means by which we must recognize disorder and disease.

"Only the vital principle thus disturbed can give to the organism its abnormal sensations and incline it to the irregular action we call disease."

To become conversant with symptoms, to judge the sphere and progress of disease by study of symptomology, is the requirement necessary for a Homeopath.

When the examination of the symptoms has been made there is no reason why one should not make a physical examination of the patient. A physician should be conversant with Anatomy and Physiology.

Be thoroughly educated in studying symptoms. The real study of sickness is the meditation of it's symptoms, and to become wise in symptoms is to become an able prescriber.

With an incurable change in a vital organ, the symptoms of disease are suppressed, as it were, by the tremendous strain on the system. This is particularly true of the malignant forms of disease results.

Therefore to manage cancer (or any other one sided chronic disease), think as follows:

1.   To cure the patient would be to cure the cancer.

2.   In order to cure the patient it is necessary to go back in his history and get those symptoms that represent the patient in a state of disease.

3.   Do not take into account the symptoms that represent the tissue in a state of disease. Such as dropsical condition, pus sacks or pain.

      If a physician cannot make a distinction between the symptoms that represent the disease per se and the symptoms that represent the result of disease he will never practice Homeopathy successfully.

4.   To think of remedies for cancer is confusion but to think remedies for the patient who appears to have cancer is orderly. Astonishing changes will take place once remedies that correspond to the conditions before the cancer began are administrated.

5.   The true morbid sensation of a healthy organ is what we must first consider.

6.   When all the strong symptoms are gathered together (with the help of patient, family and friends), the physician studying the case must separate all those things that were observed years ago from those things that are observed today, noting how have they changed and why have they changed.

LECTURE X

§ 13. Materialism in Medicine

SEVERAL paragraphs now to be read are scarcely more than a recapitulation of subjects spoken of. In going over previous paragraphs I have introduced these points in advance, because it was natural to do so in connection with the subject in hand. I will therefore glance over them until we reach something new.

"In the thirteenth paragraph Hahnemann says:

"Therefore disease (that does not come within the province of manual surgery), considered, as it is by the allopathists, as a thing separate from the living whole, from the organism and its animating vital force, and hidden in the interior, be it of ever so subtle a character, is an absurdity that could only be imagined by mind of a materialistic stamp, and has for thousands of years given to the prevailing system of medicine all those pernicious impulses that have made it a truly mischievous (non-healing) art.

The material notion referred to was that existing in the time of Hahnemann. Materialism is still growing. It seems impossible for the majority of men of the present day to perceive. Perception, that is, seeing with the understanding, seems to be entirely lost. The materialist refuses to believe anything that does not conform to the laws of time and space. It must be measured, it must be weighed, it must occupy space, or he has no idea of it, and will distinctly affirm that without this it is nothing and has no existence. Everything beyond this is to the material mind poetical, dreamy, mysterious. So they look in vain in the material world for cause. You will never find a material entity as in any way causing anything. It has no causative power, no creative influence, no propelling influence. Causes or simple substances are, in the natural state, in motion, and cause motion in the bodies that they occupy; the natural state for simple substance is that of power, of mobility, of activity. The natural state of matter is rest, quietude, silence; it has no power to move unless acted upon. Like the dead man, whose tissues are at rest, it has no action of its own. But the simple substance dominates matter and animates it.

The two worlds, the world of motion, of power, and the world of inertia, exist in one. There is a world of life and a world of dead matter are the realm of cause and the realm of result. Causes are invisible, results are visible. We see the actions of material substance, but the thinking man has only to reflect to see that these actions that are visible in material form are but result of the cause that exist in the form of simple substance which is invisible to the natural eye but visible to the spiritual eye or understanding. The materialist cannot grasp this idea, he cannot think in this way. We have the grandest confirmation of these things in the wonderful action of our potencies in the varying degrees in which they operate upon man, from the lowest to the highest. You will discover in course of time that in a large number of chronic diseases our antipsorics will cause changes in the economy, curative or otherwise, from five to seven different potencies. In this you have the demonstration of degree of simple substance, and their relation to different planes in the interior of the economy.

§ 14. There is, in the interior of man, nothing morbid that is curable, and no invisible morbid alter-

> ation that is curable, which does not make itself
> known to the accurately observing physician by
> means of morbid signs and symptoms—an
> arrangement in perfect conformity with the infinite
> goodness of the all-wise Preserver of human life.

This we have already spoken of. Every curable disease is made known to the physician by signs and symptoms. Incurable diseases have few signs and symptoms, and by their absence the disease is often thus known to be incurable. By watching the patient gradually decline without any symptoms but those which are the common expressions of pathological conditions, we see that the case is incurable and is going down to death.

All curable maladies, therefore, have signs and symptoms in order to make themselves known; their purpose is to shadow forth the disorderly condition of the vital force or interior of man, so that the physician may read it and understand its nature. This imaging forth when the human race is in a state of ignorance, or materialism, is like seeds sown upon stony ground; there is no man to understand them, to apprehend their meaning. The images of sickness are continually being formed, and only wait for a man intelligent enough to observe them, to understand their meaning to translate them, and it is possible for men, by the doctrines of homoeopathy, to become wise and intelligent enough to be conversant with these signs.

In this paragraph we also see Hahnemann's recognition of Divine Providence. It was the very recognition of Providence that enabled Hahnemann to become a man, and being directed by Divine Providence enabled him to finally perceive the law,. When his little ones were being hurled to death by strong drugs the first thought of Hahnemann was that Providence had not made these little ones to be destroyed by medicine; it seemed to him inconsistent that they should be made to take this miserable stuff. In all your experiences, if you live to be very old, you will find a very poor lot of homoeopaths among those who do not recognize Divine Order. You will find among them false science, experimentation, but never any government of principle, no thought of purpose, order or use.

Hahnemann was not in the strictest sense the discoverer of the law, for Hippocrates said that disease might be caused either by opposites or similars, but Hahnemann discovered this by pure experimentation and the following out of strict order. After reading it up he found corroboration of the principles he had discovered, and he followed along the line, growing wiser and stronger, until he formulated the code which is so simple and yet so complete. Very few are able to read the *Organon* at first and see anything in it but words, and yet the oldest practitioner of pure homoeopathy finds nothing in it to change and the older he grows and becomes more active in work the more he depends upon it and the more consistent it becomes. Although I have been teaching the *Organon* for many years, I never go over it without discovering some new thought in harmony with the general teaching. The continued study of the *Organon* bring a deeper and deeper understanding of it, because it is true.

In the 15th paragraph another thought comes up which still further shows the unit of government which we have dwelt upon so much in past lectures. Everything that flows from a center must be considered in connection with that center. Man in his healthy state is but the result of the normal activities of a unit, and he must be considered as a unit. In other words, his healthy vital force is the result of action from a center. On the other hand, when man becomes diseased in his disordered or diseased state he is still a unit and has to be considered collectively. It is not to be considered that his physiological action produces his morbid actions, but that his morbid actions so completely dominate him that he is one morbid state. This is again illustrated when he is dominated by the action of a drug (when a drug instead of a disease possesses him), then we see a morbid state, but it is still a unit of action.

There are three different subjects forming a union of study, the study of man in his natural state, the study of man in his sick state from natural disorder, and the study of man in his sick state from artificial disorder. Each remedy must be studied as a unit first and then those units may be compared. To intermingle comparative Materia Medica without a full knowledge of units is a mistake. This I have found out by experience in my earlier teaching. I have taught much comparative Materia Medica, thinking that a wise course to pursue, but have since abandoned that plan and now study each remedy as a unit, just as I advise the study of each disease as a unit. When one remedy is fully mastered, or one disease is fully mastered, then you are ready to compare. First of all think of measles as measles, and whooping cough as whooping cough, and, when you come to the chronic diseases, ascertain all the things that have been observed in syphilis, and all the symptoms that have been observed in sycosis, and all those that have been observed in psora. You are then prepared to enter the study of the Materia Medica and see the relationship of some remedies to the acute miasms and the relationship of other remedies to the chronic miasms. You will see particularly the image of measles in some remedies, the image of whooping cough in other, and the image of psora, syphilis and sycosis in others. Then you are ready to proceed with what may be called individualization, because these are the most general, and from these we go into particulars and then into comparison. This is the classical way to proceed, and when it is followed the physician becomes wise and intelligent and can apply the Materia Medica with wonderful precision. Such was Hahnemann's method.

Classroom Notes

Materialism in Medicine

1. Simple Substance are in motion in their natural state and cause motion in bodies that they occupy.

2. The natural state for simple substance is that of power, of mobility and of activity.

3. The natural state of matter is of rest, quietude and of silence. It has no power to move unless acted upon.

4.   The simple substances dominates matter and animates it.

5.   The two worlds, the world of motion, i.e. of power; and the world of inertia exists in one.

6.   The world of motion is the world of life, the realm of thought, the realm of simple substances, the realm of causes.

7.   The world of matter is the realm of inertia, realm of results, realm of ultimates.

8.   Causes are invisible and results are visible.

9.   Every curable disease is made known to the physician by signs and symptoms.

10. Incurable disease have few signs and symptoms and by there absence the disease is thus known to be incurable.

Man in his healthy state is but his result of the normal activities of a unit, and he must be considered as unit (the mind and the body as one unit.)

On the other hand when man is diseased, in his disordered or diseased state he is still a unit and this diseased unit has to be considered collectively. Therefore three different subjects form a union of study of disease in human economy:

1.   The study of man in its natural state.

2.   The study of man in his sick state from natural disorder.

3.   The study of man in his sick state from the artificial disorder.

LECTURE XI

§ 16. (1) Healthy State. (2) How made Sick. (3) How Cured. Only Deranged and Cured in Dynamic Planes

§ 16. Our vital force, as a spirit-like dynamis, cannot be attacked and infected by injurious influences on the healthy organism caused by the external inimical forces that disturb the harmonious play of life otherwise than in a spirit-like (dynamic) way, and in like manner all such morbid derangements (diseases) cannot be removed from it by the physician in any other way than by the spirit-like (dynamic, virtual), alternative powers of the serviceable medicines acting upon our spirit-like vital force, which preserves them through the medium of the sentient faculty of the nerves everywhere present in the organism, so that it is only by their dynamic action of the vital force that remedies are able to re-establish and do actually re-establish health and vital harmony *after* the changes in the health of the patient cognizable by our senses (the totality of the symptoms) have revealed the disease to the carefully observing and investigating physician as fully as was requisite in order to enable him to cure it.

THE 16th paragraph furnishes the subject that we will talk about this morning. It treats of three states: (1) of the state of health, or the normal activities of the body, (2) of how that state is made sick or turned into disorder, and (3) of how that disordered state can be turned into health. If we could find a man in a state of perfect health, we might subject him to shock, to injuries, to the actions of the cruder things around us, and he would pass through them or they would pass away without leaving upon him any such thing as a disorder. He might be under the influence of that shock a short time, but when reaction came, if it came at all, it would leave him free from miasm, he would not have therefrom either an acute or chronic disease. It is only by the action of immaterial substances, simple substances acting upon a plane similar to the plane of his susceptibility, that he can become infected with a sickness; that is, the resultant action of a substance capable of operating from his innermost to his outermost, and establishing evidence which we call symptoms. If the outermost alone is acted upon the vital force of the man is only temporarily disturbed, but there is not established a definite disorder (not even a limited one) that can run a course with a beginning, a period of progress and decline, such as the miasms do.

Whatever depresses the tissues of man, or his bodily functions, only acts temporarily, and is not capable of establishing a true disease. Take, for instance, the cruder drugs that we see used as a physic. You may give the patient the coarser and cruder forms of drugs as purgatives and emetics, and he will go through the shock and return to his original state. It is only after the most violent and long continued use of liquids that there can be implanted upon him a drug disease, and even that is largely superficial in comparison to a natural diseased condition. The constant use of Bromide of Potassium will produce effects in time, but that drug does not go to the depths, it operates upon the tissues, producing a coarser form of disease, but not miasmatic in character. Take also the coarser poisons as an example. Many of them can be taken into the stomach in crude form with very little manifestation upon the vital force, indeed the more active and virulent and condensed the poison the smaller the collective symptoms image. The small pox crust can be swallowed and it will be digested and very little trouble come from it, but the inhalation of the atmosphere that contains the aura of smallpox upon a place corresponding to the susceptibility of the individual will bring him down with the disease having a definite prodrome, a period of progress and a period of decline, showing that the very foundation of the man's nature has been struck. Such an operation is upon the internals of man upon his invisible, immaterial substance, and it operates from within out, producing ultimates in his tissues, establishing results upon the skin.

Hahnemann in this paragraph affirms that nothing, except in the form of a simple substance, can so implant itself upon the economy as to run its course as a disease either acute or chronic. No disease can implant itself upon the economy through its ultimate forms; only in its invisible forms can it so act. All disease known to man are in the form of simple substance, an invisible something that cannot be detected by the chemist or the microscopist, and will never be detected in the natural world. Disease cause is known, and known only, from its effects; it is not capable of investigation by the natural senses and can only be investigated as to its results. Everything that can be seen, felt or observed, or detected with the microscope, is but an ultimate, a result. It is only by the understanding, by reasoning from first to last and then back again, that we can perceive that disease causes are invisible.

The body can be affected, the tissues can be affected, and ultimates can be affected by ultimates, there can be friction between ultimates; things in this world can collide with other things in this world and they may destroy each other; ultimates may destroy ultimates; but such a thing as disease occurring in ultimates except through dynamic changes is impossible.

Nor can any agency which is an ultimate act upon the human economy curatively, turning into vital order the innermost of *life*. Vital disorder cannot be turned into order except by something similar in quality to the vital force. It is not similitude in quantity that we want, in weights and measures, but it is similarity in quality, in power, in plane, that must be sought for.

Medicines, therefore, cannot affect the high and interior planes of the physical economy unless they are raised to the plane of similarity in quality. The individual who needs Sulphur in the very highest degrees may take Sulphur sufficient to move his bowels, may rub it upon the skin, may wear it in his stockings, can take Sulphur baths, all without effect upon his disease. In that form the drug is not in correspondence with his sickness. It does not affect him in the same plane in which he is sick, and so it cannot affect the cause and flow from thence to the circumference. So with all the coarser drugs, they do not cure. We sometimes see the outermost effects of disease, disease located in the outer planes, temporarily removed by the lower potencies and crude drugs, but it is only as to the exteriors and ultimates that the cure is effected, and as it does not reach the innermost degrees it is not permanent. In acute diseases also crude drugs sometimes accomplish their purpose, because the outermost which they affect is only on the surface and the innermost has, in acute disease, the tendency to go away of itself; if his life can simply be spared until the disease has run its course the patient will recover. But the chronic miasms are only reached as to their ultimate symptoms, and these are caused to subside only temporarily or are suppressed by the action of the crude or ultimate forms of medicine.

I look back upon the time when my own mind was in a cloud as to this subject, and if I refer to it here it may be of use to you. I remember when I first read from Hahnemann that potentized medicines would cure the sick that it seemed to me a mystery. I had no knowledge upon which to found belief in such things. I began to practice with the lower potencies and with crude drugs in attempting to carry out the law, but with these means I was able to cure only superficial complaints. My work was far from satis: factory, yet it was somewhat better than the old things, it was milder than physicking and purging and emesis. Of course I rested upon my opinions and belief for my knowledge; everyone does that.

Later I resolved to test the 30th potency to see if there was not yet medicine in it, and I prepared with my own hands the 30th potency of Podophyllum with water on the centesimal scale, after the fashion of Hahnemann, having been told that water was as good as alcohol and it was only the attenuation that was required. This was during an epidemic of diarrhoea that looked like Podophyllum, but I had not the courage to give the 30th and still continued to use my stronger medicines. One day a child was brought into my office in the mother's arms. She brought it in hastily, and it did not seem as if it could live long. It was an infant, and while it lay in her arms a thin yellowish fecal stool ran over my carpet. The odor struck me as like that I had been reading about as the odor of the Podophyllum stool; it was horribly offensive, stinking and the stool was so copious that the mother made remark that she did not know where it all came from. I said to myself, this is a case upon which to test Hahnemann's 30th potency. So I fixed up some of the Podophyllum 30 and put it on the child's tongue, and sent the mother home, fearing that the child would soon die, as it was very ill, face pinched and drawn, cadaveric, and had a dreadful odor about it. Next morning when making my rounds I had to pass the house. I expected to see crepe on the door. I did not dare to call, though I was very much worried about it, so I drove past; but there was no crepe on the door. I drove home again that way, although it was quite a distance out of the way, and still there was no crepe on the door; but standing in the door way was the grandmother, who said: "Doctor, the baby is all right this morning." Then I began to feel better, thinking I had not killed it. Perhaps some of you have been in the same state of mind.

That little child did not need any more medicine. After that I had quite a number of Podophyllum cases, and the 30th did the work to my astonishment. It was different from anything I had ever seen; the cures were almost instantaneous, it seemed as if there would be no more stool after the first dose of medicine. I did not always give the single dose. I used that 30th all the season, and then made up my mind that if the 30th of Podophyllum was good other 30th would also be, and I ought to have as many of them as possible. I made a good many 30ths by hand, and finally succeeded in making up one hundred and twenty-six remedies, some of them in the 200th potency, and these I used. Then I procured a set of 200ths and higher and practiced with them. I followed on in this way and in a few years I discovered that by giving higher and higher potencies the remedies seemed to operate more and more interiorly.

I found that a chronic case that would be relieved by moderately high potencies would only improve for a matter of weeks, but on the administration of much higher potencies the work would be taken up, and in that way the same patient could be carried on from one potency to another. If I give you the conversation of one patient with me from time to time you may understand better what I mean. I saw this patient for the first time some fifteen years ago, when he was stoop-shouldered and had a fairly phthisical aspect. He had a catarrhal state of the chest, and it looked as though it might end in phthisis. On his symptoms he received Sulphur about 6 m. He was violently aggravated by this dose of medicine all his symptoms were made worse, and he came back to the office saying that the medicine had made him sick. I had attained knowledge of the aggravation from a similar remedy, so I gave him sugar. At the end of another week he came back and told me he was better, much better, that he did not want me to give him any more of that first medicine, but he wanted more of the last, as it had made him so much better. So I kept him on the medicine which pleased him for a period of probably six or seven weeks. One time he returned and told me he did not want that last medicine, but he wanted that medicine that helped him so. By that I know enough to give him another dose of Sulphur. Within the next day or two he ran in and said, "You young rascal, you gave me that medicine that made me sick in the first place," so he got sugar again and went on this time for five or six weeks, or perhaps longer. Then he came back again saying, "Now, I do not think you understand me, for I am having my old symptoms back. I wish you would study my case again." So I went all over his case and he got another dose of Sulphur 6 m. He reported this time, " Well, I do not feel any better; I am just about the same." He was not stirred up this time, you see. I waited a little longer and saw no relief from the last dose.

Here are all the symptoms calling for Sulphur, shall I give him crude Sulphur? I cannot give remedy that is not indicated. The experience of the older men says "go higher." I gave him Sulphur 55 m., and in a few days he came back upon me, saying, "You rascal, you gave me that first medicine again. I do not want that stuff." Finally I got him cooled down, gave him some sugar and assured him that he would be better in a few days, and he went on for six or seven weeks with great improvement. After a while I explained to him that when the remedy did not act I had to give him something to stir him up. Of course I did not say anything to him about sugar.

When you have learned what your medicines will do it is a good thing to say to the patient, "Do not be alarmed or astonished when such and such things happen." Otherwise they will get alarmed and go off and perhaps get another doctor. The 55 m. of Sulphur relieved that patient in a couple of doses, far apart, and then ceased to relieve him any more. Next he received the c.m. which worked just as the other potencies had done, and finally he got to the mm. Which acted just like the c.m., and from that potency he went on being restored to health. When you see these things you have a confirmation in them of the doctrines of the law. Experience does not lead to these things, but principles which thereafter are confirmed by experience. When a patient has been carried up through a series of potencies he will often remain unaffected by that remedy in a lower realm of potency or in the crude, unless he is overwhelmingly dosed by it, and then he will be poisoned.

The third proposition in this paragraph is that medicines will not act curatively, or in a way to turn the body into order and turn off disease, unless potentized to correspond to the degrees in which the man is sick. Such as are sick in a middle plane are sick from that plane to the outermost. Such as are sick in the interior planes are sick throughout to the outermost. When the disorder is in the very depth of his physical nature then it is in the form of chronic disease; *i.e.,* all there is of him is sick, and of such there is no tendency to recovery but a continued progress. Such is the order of psora, syphilis and sycosis.

The nutritive plane is entirely in the outermost, that is, in the tissues. Assimilation goes on in the tissues. It is simply in the realm of tissues and ultimates that crude drugs operate; they can only disturb ultimates, and the inharmonious condition is the inharmony of ultimates, the outermost plane. Of course, if the outermost of the physical is disturbed the whole economy suffers, and the body ceases to furnish a good instrument to be operated upon by the powers within; but a *true disease,* with periods of prodrome, progress and decline or continuance, cannot be implanted upon the economy except it be by a dynamic cause. And hence necessarily man cannot be cured except by drugs attenuated until they have become similar to the nature or quality of disease cause. Disease cause and the disease-curing drug must be similar in nature; unlike causes would not produce like effects. We can arrive at similar causes by studying the effects that are similar. When we examine into a case and find a certain group of symptoms and in the effects produced by a certain drug we see like symptoms, we have a right to presume that the quality or nature in both is similar. The causes must be similar if the effects are similar in nature and quality. When the physician goes out the bedside he asks himself, Do I know a remedy that has produced upon a healthy man, symptoms like these? He must pass judgment upon the symptoms, he must be an artist in application and capable of discerning the finer shades of difference and similitude.

Classroom Notes

Sickness and cure on Dynamic Plane

Man is only deranged and cured in dynamic planes:

1.   Hahnemann in this paragraph affirms that nothing except in the form of simple substance, can so implant itself upon the internal state so as to turn its course into a disease (acute or chronic).

2.   Vital disorder cannot be converted back into order expect by something similar in quality to the vital force.

3.   It is not similitude in quantity that we want, in weight and measures but it is similarity in quality, in power, in plane, that must be sought for [medicines should be selected on the basis of totality (quality) and the dose should be selected on the basis of vitality (power)].

4.   Potency should be selected on the basis of plane of activity desired.

Crude medicines therefore cannot change the high and interior planes of the physical economy unless they are raised to the plane of similarity in quality.

By giving higher and highest potencies the remedies seem to operate more and more interiorly. It is only in the realm of tissues and ultimates that the crude drugs operate.

LECTURE XII

The Removal of the Totality of Symptoms Means the Removal of the Cause

---

§ 17. Now, as in the cure effected by the removal of the whole of the perceptible signs and symptoms of the disease the internal alteration of the vital force to which the disease is due—consequently the whole of the disease—is at the same time removed, it follows that the physician has only to remove the whole of the symptoms in order, at the same time, to abrogate and annihilate the internal change, that is to say, the morbid derangement of the vital force—consequently the totality of the disease, *the disease itself*. But when the disease is annihilated the health is restored, and this is the highest, the sole aim of the physician who knows the true object of his mission, which consists not in learned-sounding prating but in giving aid to the sick

---

THE idea of this paragraph is that the removal of the totality of the symptoms is actually the removal of the cause. It may not be

known that causes are continued into effects (*i.e.*, that causes continue in ultimates), but it is true that all ultimates to a great extent
contain the cause of the beginnings. And since cause continues
into ultimates and things in ultimates shadow forth cause, the
removal of all the symptoms will lead any rational man to assume
that the cause has been removed. This will lead you to see that if
a large number of symptoms manifest themselves through a diseased ovary, and that ovary is removed, the cause of the symptoms has not been removed and will manifest through some other
part of the body, perhaps the other ovary or some organ that is
weak.

It is a serious matter to remove any organ through which disease is manifested. When there are two or more of these pathological conditions established upon the body and one is removed the
other immediately becomes worse. For instance, if there is a
structural change in the knee joint and the surgeon removes the
knee, while there is a corresponding structural change in the kidneys or liver which he cannot remove, the latter immediately
becomes worse and breaks down as soon as the knee joint is
removed. In the same way we find in a tuberculosis condition of
the lungs that it may remain in a very quiet state so long as a fis-
tula *in ano* keeps on discharging but the allopath comes along and
closes that vent and immediately there is a cropping out of the disease by infiltration of the lungs and the patient comes to an early
death. The results of diseases are necessary in many instances.
Sometimes these results are tuberculous conditions, which are the
ultimate outcome or effects from cause, and contain at times the
seeds of beginnings of a similar kind. They are not themselves
beginnings, yet they contain causes. Unless causes are removed
from beginning to end the disease can reproduce itself. This
includes the first proposition of Hahnemann as to the cure of disease, which means permanent removal of the totality of the symptoms, thus removing the cause and turning disorder into order, and
as a consequence the results of disease are removed. The totality
cannot be removed without removing the cause.

"But when the disease is annihilated the health is restored; and this is the highest, the sole aim of the physician who knows the true object of his mission, which consists not in learned-sounding prating but in giving aid to the sick." Hahnemann gives this warning note against discoursing dogmatically upon the flimsy theories of man. It was the custom in Hahnemann's time for men to cloak their ignorance in technicalities; that is, to use technicalities for the purpose of appearing wise. It is done at the present day, I have heard physicians talk to simple-minded people in technicalities. Wise people seldom use technicalities. There is nothing in this world to becloud the understanding as to deal in technicalities, they are cramped and often meaningless. The doctrines of homoeopathy should not be clouded in technicalities, but should be considered and talked out in the simplest forms of speech. When talking of the *Organon* and its doctrines, talk good English, if you are English, and use simple forms of speech. One technical word will sometimes mean a whole sentence, and can be constituted to mean a good many different things. Technicalities are a sort of scapegoat to carry off the sins of our ignorance.

The "totality of the symptoms" means a good deal. It is a wonderfully broad thing. It may be considered to be all that is essential of the disease. It is all that is visible and represents the disease in the natural world to the eye, the touch and external understanding of man. It is all that enables the physician to individualize between diseases and between remedies; the entire representation of a disease is the totality of the symptoms, and the entire representation of a drug is the totality of the symptoms. It does not mean the little independent symptoms, but it means that which will bring to the mind a clear idea of the nature of the sickness. Many of the little symptoms that occur can be left out of the total without marring, but the essence, the characteristics, the image must be there, as that is of importance to the physician, being to him the sole indication in the choice of the remedy. It is true that the old prescriber may be able to perceive the totality if he can see only a small portion of it. Prescribing in that way, however, is very often a mistake, for when that which was wanting is brought out the physician sees that he has prescribed only for the side view, as it were. You become well acquainted with old friends and know them by even a partial view or by the gait, or voice, but it is not so with strangers. Strangers have to be studied, criticized and examined. It requires a long time to know the stranger's methods, to find out how he performs his business, whether he is cheerful or not, to know the character, to know the man. So it is with the totality of the symptoms, for to a great extent every sickness is a new sickness. If the patient has nothing to conceal he will delineate his symptoms cheerfully, but if he has something to conceal it becomes a hard matter to obtain the totality of his symptoms. But this totality must be obtained, for there is no other means of ascertaining the nature of the remedy that he is in need of, as it is expressed in the eighteenth paragraph:

From this indubitable truth, that besides the totality
of the symptoms, nothing can be any means be
discovered in diseases wherewith they could
express their need of aid, it follows undeniably that
the sum of all the symptoms in each individual
case of disease must be the *sole indication,* the
sole guide to direct us in the choice of a remedy.

But it is not enough to consider the totality as a grand whole; besides considering all the symptoms collectively each individual symptom must be considered. Every symptom must be examined to see what relation it sustains to and what position it fills in that totality in order that we may know its value, whether it is a common symptom, whether it is a particular symptom, or whether a peculiarly characteristic symptom. This we shall consider later in course.

---

§ 19. Now, as diseases are nothing more than *alter-
ations in the state of health of the healthy individual*
which express themselves by morbid signs, and the
cure is only possible by a *change to the healthy
condition of the state of health of the diseased*

individual, it is very evident that medicines could
never cure diseases if they did not possess the
power of altering man's state of health, which
depends on sensations and function; indeed that
their curative power must be owing *solely* to this
power they possess of altering man's state of health.

The statement is that medicines must be capable of effecting
changes in the economy or they cannot restore order in the economy. If the medicine is too high to effect a disturbance in an irregularly governed economy it will be too high to effect a cure in that
economy. The potency must be consistent with the degree of susceptibility that calls for the medicine. This susceptibility includes
a wide range of potency, so that from the 30th to the cm. there is
seldom a miss in actual experience. It is seldom that the potency
is too high, but that it is higher than is necessary is often true. No
drug can act curatively except by its ability to effect changes, and
it is known that drugs do effect changes by their provings; but in
the provings the drug has been increased in quantity or reduced in
quality in accordance with the judgment of the prover. Many
times the coarser substances effect few changes and sometimes
none, whereas the higher substances make sick; this is in accordance with the state of susceptibility. Some provers are susceptible to the higher who are not at all susceptible to the lower. There
are patients who are not in the least susceptible to a single drop of
tincture of Coffea but who are extremely susceptible to the higher potencies of Coffea. Such patients, however, are often made
sick by large quantities of coffee. Lycopodium in its crude form
has upon most people no effect, but in the higher potencies is
capable, if followed up continuously, of affecting almost everyone. The effect that medicines have upon the sick in restoring
order can best be observed by inducing the effects upon healthy
individuals, which we call *proving.*

You might easily suppose, by the way the modern firms bring
their medicines before us, that they have by a great effort of their
will, and by great meditation, thought out what these drugs will

do to the human family. For the purpose of ascertaining the state of medicine at the present time I very often listen patiently to a drummer from some of the New York houses. He will speak his piece, tell what this wonderful combination will do, how many diseases it will cure, and then I ask him how he finds this out. "Oh, the doctors say so. Here are the testimonials." "But how do they find it out?" "Oh, they use them."

But the drugs have not been proved, and their use is not in accordance with what the homoeopathy knows the drugs will produce or cure. If you go into a friendly drug store and talk with the druggist you will find these medicines which have been concocted in the prescriptions of all the fashionable doctors in the neighbourhood. In six months from that time if you go to that same store you will not find one of those drugs in use, but a new set following the visit of the traveling man who has come around to represent their wonderful properties. Do not think that I refer entirely to the old school, because a large percentage of these prescriptions is from professed homoeopaths, and that is as much homoeopathy as anything they do. The majority of homoeopaths do these things, attempting to establish a homoeopathic practice upon an allopathic foundation. They try to become fashionable and change their prescriptions as the ladies change their bonnets with the season.

In § 20. Hahnemann says:

This spirit-like power to alter man's state of health (and hence to cure diseases) which lies hidden in the inner nature of medicines can never be discovered by us by a mere effort of reason; it is only by experience of the phenomena it displays when acting in the state of health of man that we can become clearly cognizant of it.

There is only one way of finding out what Aconite will do to the economy, and that is to give it to many men and note the symptoms that these men experience as the manifestations of Aconite. It is first necessary to know that drugs can make man

Aconite. It is first necessary to know that drugs can make man sick, and next to know what that state of sickness is. Every medicine that a homoeopath uses should have been thoroughly proven upon the healthy so that its symptoms image shall have been thoroughly brought out. It is a burning shame upon the homoeopathic profession that so large a number of drugs exist in the homoeopathic pharmacies, and that these drugs are recommended for such and such diseases without any investigation as to their properties, other than perhaps that doctor so-and-so, on the recommendation of some old woman, has used this or that drug for dropsy. Such as thing is positively condemned in every line of the *Organon* and by every doctrine. There is no principle in it, it is unscientific, and unworthy of the vocation of a doctor. Every drug must be thoroughly proven upon the healthy. In our study of the Materia Medica I do not encumber you with partially proved drugs. We can study these after we have studied those that have been well proved. The "Guiding Symptoms" contain many medicines only partially proven and it is often a matter of accident when cures are made with them. But the old remedies that have been handed down from the masters, and that have had years of trial, come to us as friends which can learn of and become acquainted with. You cannot become acquainted with unproved drugs. When books tell you that a drug is good for this or that, pay no attention to them, but when a book tells you that a drug has produced such and such symptoms study these; that is a piece of valuable information. The old school Materia Medica is made up of the results of medicine upon sickness, an unscientific guide, a fluctuating scale.

Classroom Notes

Causes, Symptoms and Cure

Removal of the totality of the symptoms means the removal of the cause (internal fundamental cause).

[Para: 17]
Since causes continue in ultimates (results). The removal of all the symptoms (the symptoms being the ultimate expression of the disordered interior) will lead any rational man to assume that the cause has been removed from the disordered interior.

[Para: 18]
The totality of symptoms means a good deal. It is a wonderfully broad thing. Many of the little symptoms that a patient relates can be left out of the totality without marring, but the essence, the characteristics, the image, of the disease must be there. As these are important to the physician, being to him the sole indication in the choice of remedy.

[Para: 19]
1.   Potency must be consistent with the degree of susceptibility that calls for the medicine. This susceptibility includes a wide range of potency [From 30 C to CM]
2.   If the medicine is too high to cause a disturbance in an irregularly governed internal state, it will be too high to facilitate a cure in that economy.
3.   Many times the coarser substances effect few changes and sometimes none, whereas the higher substances make sick. This is in accordance with the state of susceptibility.

[Para: 20]
It is necessary first, to know that drugs can make man sick and then to know what that state of sickness is.

Every medicine that a Homeopath uses should be thoroughly proven upon the healthy so that its symptom image is brought out as regard to its characteristics and peculiarities. Only then its essence can be clearly perceived.

LECTURE XIII

§ 21-25. The law of Similars

In these paragraphs Hahnemann summarizes what he has said before and points out the necessary conclusions. In doing so he proves that the only method of applying medicines profitably in disease is the homoeopathic method. We daily see that the antipathic and heteropathic methods have no tendency of permanency in their results. By these means there are effected changes in the economy and changes in the symptoms but no permanent cure, the tendency being simply to the establishment of another disease, often worse than the first, and without eradicating the first. In this connection we might speak of the giving of morphine and purgatives. The friends of the patient plead with you to stop the pain or give something to move the bowels for the relief of the patient. You know quite well that the relief from morphine is very transient, but when you are occupying the ground of principle there is the strongest reason why a dose of morphine should never be administered. After giving morphine changes are observed which are really detrimental to the patient. The symptoms are changed, and this is always unfortunate. The same objection applies to the giving of chloroform in labor. No woman at the present day is well enough to go through labor without some symptoms calling for a remedy. Hence, if you give chloroform in labor, you put your patient in a state in which she is unable to express the symptoms of her own condition. If, at the close of labor, she was about to give forth symptoms that would indicate to the intelligent physician what remedy she needed (perhaps to overcome a life-time of suffering) you would be deprived of knowing what the remedy was by this act of foolishness.

---

§ 26. This depends on the following homoeopathic law of nature which was sometimes, indeed, vaguely surmised but not hitherto fully recognized, and to what is due every real cure that has ever taken place: *A weaker dynamic affection is permanently extinguished in the living organism by a stronger one, if the latter (whilst differing in kind), is very similar to the former in its manifestation.*

In this paragraph Hahnemann distinctly declares that the phenomena of cure depend entirely upon fixed law, the law of similars or the law that governs homoeopathy. After Hahnemann had made a number of provings he gathered together from the literature a great number of reported cures for the purpose of observing whether the cures had been made accidentally or from purpose and whether they were in accordance with the law of similars or with the principle of dissimilars In every instance he was able to see that the cures had been made in accordance with the law of similars, viz., that the drug which cured in each case was capable of producing symptoms similar to those which it cured. This is true in all planes, under all circumstances, and all other apparent cures are not cures but suppressions.

"A dynamic disease in the living economy of man is extinguished in a permanent manner by another that is more powerful when the latter (without being of the same species) bears a strong resemblance to it in its mode of manifesting itself." That sentence seemed to be about the best way of expressing the law in Hahnemann's time. The words "more powerful," or more intense, would afford a natural way of expressing it, but when one has lived in homoeopathy, and has been able to perceive its inner workings, the word "powerful" expresses a different thought. If we follow along the line of potentization we lose the idea of power that is manifest to an uninitiated mind. We enter the world of thought and, therein learn of a different kind of power or intensity. When we think naturally of power or intensity the mind is at once carried to the idea of intensity as in an electrical problem in which we increase the intensity by increasing the number of batteries. On the other hand, Hahnemann's expression leads to the idea of intensity, having qualities more internal, higher, prior; i.e., in the sense of from first to last, the more internal it is the more intense, the more it approaches the first substance, so that intensity as to cause means higher or more internal, higher in the sense of subtleness or fineness.

The word "powerful" then, you will please note, contains an interior thought, and that is the only way to bring the mind to realize what is meant. Powerful is actually from within and hence we potentize, going higher and higher, in order that we may reach intensity, and it is in this sense that the remedy becomes more powerful by potentization. As a matter of fact, when speaking upon the material plane, the remedy grows weaker by potentization because the material is actually reduced. It would seem strange to a materialist, to an old school doctor for instance, who has not thought of anything but the giving of great pills, to say that Aconite becomes more powerful by being attenuated. To him it would just be saying that it becomes more powerful the weaker it becomes and yet it is really so, though he cannot see it.

"A dynamic disease is extinguished by another that is more powerful when the latter is similar to it." The first proposition is that it must be similar and then it must be intense enough. The more there is in the interior, the more there to expect in the exterior. So it is with the light of the sun. it is grander than all other lights, because there is more in its interior; it is purer, it is more dynamical and it will turn aside and destroy all other light.

This law of similars is seen prominently in the natural world.

We see it from man to man. It is easily illustrated among the insane. It is the secret of mind cure, and there are many instances of mind cure that are based on the law of similars. One example of this is seen in the young girl who has lost her mother or lover and is ill as a consequence, is depressed with grief, is constantly sobbing, and has become melancholy. She sits in a corner, hears nobody, thinks no one can pity her because no one has had just such grief. Let us apply allopathic treatment to her. "Come, there is nothing the matter with you; why don't you brace yourself up; why don't you try to arouse yourself?" But this only throws her into a deeper state of melancholy. Scolding and harsh treatment do no good. But introduce the homoeopathic treatment, employ a nurse if you will who is a good actress and who has gone through the same identical grief, and let her make a big fuss in the other corner. Pretty soon the patient will say, "You seem to have the same grief that I have." "Yes, I have lost a lover." "Well, you can sympathize with me," and the two fall to bellowing and weep it out together. There is a bond of sympathy. Sometimes a curable case of insanity can be reached in this way, and thus we have a mind cure. Hahnemann made use of this plan in curing insanity. When a patient would exert her will, but is unable on account of the physical encumbrances, then the homoeopathic remedy will restore order.

---

§ 27. The curative power of medicines, therefore depends on their symptoms, similar to the disease but superior to it in strength, so that each individual case of disease is most surely, radically, rapidly and permanently annihilated and removed only by a medicine capable of producing (in the human system) in the most similar and complete manner the totality of its symptoms, which at the same time are stronger than the disease.

Then it is not sufficient merely to give the drug itself regardless of its form. It is not sufficient to give the crude drug, but the plane upon which it is to be given is a question of study. The attenuation also must be similar to the disease cause. In a proving the crude drug may bring forth a mass of symptoms in one prover, but when a person is sick those symptoms will not be touched by the crude drug because the patient does not sustain the similar relation or susceptibility that the one did who proved it.

In paragraph 29, Hahnemann has given an explanation of the law of cure. He himself preludes it by saying that he does not attach much importance to it. You are not in any way bound to consider it, and it is usually omitted in this course.

Classroom Notes

The Law of Similars

[Para: 26]
Please take note the word 'Stronger' and \ 'Powerful', contain an interior thought.

Powerful is actually from within and hence we potentise, going higher and higher in order that we may reach some intensity and it is this sense that the remedy become more powerful by potentisation.

As a matter of fact upon the material plane, the remedy grows weaker by potentisation because the material is actually reduced.

[Para: 27]
It is not sufficient merely to give the drug itself regardless of its form.

It is the **plane** *upon which it is to be given is a question of study. The potency must also be similar to the plane of the cause of disease.*

LECTURE XIV

§ 30, ECT. Susceptibility

§ 30. The human body appears to admit of being much more powerfully affected in it health by medicines (partly because we have the regulation of the dose in our own power) than by natural morbid stimuli—for natural diseases are cured and overcome by suitable medicines.

§ 31. The inimical forces, partly psychical, partly physical, to which our terrestrial existence is exposed, which are termed morbific noxious agents, do not possess the power of morbidly deranging the health of man unconditionally; but we are made ill by them only when our organism is sufficiently disposed and susceptible to the attack of the morbific cause that may be present and to be altered in its health, deranged and made to undergo abnormal sensations and functions, hence they do not produce disease in everyone, nor at all times.

§ 32. But it is quite otherwise with the artifical morbific agents which we term medicines. Every real medicine, namely, acts at *all* times, under *all* circumstances, on *every* living human being, and produces in him its peculiar symptoms (distinctly perceptible if the dose be large enough) so that evidently every human organism is liable to be affected, and, as it were, inoculated with the

> medical disease, at all times and absolutely (uncon-
> ditionally), which, as before said, is by no means
> the case with the natural disease.

INCIDENTALLY these paragraphs have a bearing upon degree or intensity (which is potentization), upon the repetition of the dose, and upon susceptibility, things which must be known by the homoeopathic physician in order that he may be a good prescriber. We have studied potentization sufficiently to see that disease causes exist among attenuated things, the infinitesimal or immaterial substances, and thus the physician must see that the curative remedy must be on the same plane. He must know why it is that he should give but one dose, and the rationale by which susceptibility is satisfied.

In contagion (and consequently in cure) there is practically but one dose administered, or at least that which is sufficient to cause a suspension of influx. When cause ceases to flow in a particular direction it is because resistance is offered for causes flow only in the direction of least resistance and so when resistance appears influx ceases, the cause no longer flows in. Now in the beginning of disease, *i.e.*, in the stage of contagion, there is this limit to influx, for if man continued to receive the cause of disease (if there were no limits to its influx) he would receive enough to kill him, for it would run a continuous course until death. But when susceptibility is satisfied, there is a cessation of cause, and when cause ceases to flow into ultimates, not only do the ultimates cease but cause itself has already ceased.

Hahnemann states that we have more power over human beings with drugs than disease cause, for man is only susceptible to natural diseases upon a certain plane. Disease causes, existing as they do as immaterial substances, flow into man in spite of him; he can neither control nor resist them, and they make him sick. But certain changes occur and man ceases to be susceptible, and there is no longer an inflowing of cause into his economy; a suspension has taken place, because susceptibility has ceased. Susceptibility ceases when changes occur in the economy that bar out any more influx.

But cure and contagion are very similar, and the principles applying to one apply to the other. There is this difference: in cure we have the advantage of change of potency, and this enables us to suit the varying susceptibilities of sick man. Because of these varying degrees of susceptibility some are protected from disease cause and some are made sick; the one who is made sick is susceptible to the disease cause in accordance with the plane he is in and the degree of attenuation that happens to be present at the time of contagion. The degree of the disease cause fits his susceptibility at the moment he is made sick. But it is not so with medicines. Man has all the degrees of potentization, and by these he can make changes and thereby fit the medicine to the varying susceptibility of man in varying qualities or degrees. Hence Hahnemann writes, "Medicines (particularly as it depends on us to vary doses according to our will) appear to have greater power in affecting the state of health than the natural morbific irritation, for natural diseases are cured and subdued by appropriate medicines."

Now, here we might ask the question, when does a medicine that has been administered cease to be homoeopathic? The same principle as to susceptibility must apply, because of the similarity between cure and contagion. Let me illustrate it in this way. Suppose we have a case of diphtheria, and after due study Lachesis appears to be the most similar of all medicines and a dose is given. Now, when does Lachesis cease to be homoeopathic? When the symptoms that indicated it change, then it is no longer indicated. If it is given at all after this change, it operates upon a different plane from what it did in its homoeopathicity, and if it acts at all it does not act curatively but depressingly. Any more than just enough to supply the susceptibility is a surplus and is dangerous. In a chronic disease administer Sulphur when it is clearly indicated, and the symptoms disappear and the patient feels better. Then the remedy ceases to be homoeopathic, and if it is administered longer whatever action it has, is neither homoeopathic nor desirable.

But man argues if a little will do good, more will do more good. Enough to effect change is all that can be homoeopathic; when certain changes are effected then the physician must wait.

Enough medicine must be given to establish order, and that is done almost instantaneously; at most it is but a matter of a few hours, and as long as order continues after it has once begun, so long "hands off." That is just the way contagion takes place. In diphtheria the disease begins, susceptibility ceases, a change takes place that protects the man from any further disease cause flowing into the body, and the disease develops and manifests itself by its symptoms.

The repetition of dose is advised by many wise heads, but if we understand this doctrine it will be clear to us that such repetition of dose is perfectly useless. It is true, that in vigorous, robust subjects who have lightning-like reaction the dose may be repeated and changes occur for the better if the remedy is not quite homoeopathic to the case. But some are injured in this way because they are delicate subjects, whose reaction is slow; the reaction is actually prevented by the repetition of the dose; *i.e.*, the order we have tried to establish is actually prevented. Hahnemann teaches that the human economy is more under control of man than under the control of disease, for the economy can be affected only by such disease as it is susceptible to, but man, whether for the purpose of proving or for the purpose of curing, can so vary the dose that he can always get results, and the very susceptible ones are terribly damaged by the repetition of the dose.

In the thirty-first paragraph Hahnemann says that disease causes are limited in their ability to effect changes in health, to certain conditions and states; *i.e.*, to susceptibility. This is all Hahnemann says of this doctrine of cessation of cause after certain evolutions have taken place. We see that when a natural disease is taken it runs its period, and tends to decline, and the patient will not be susceptible until another change of state has arrived. It is not true that man will go out of one state of susceptibility to a disease, and in a few days go into another state of susceptibility to that same disease. There must be a change, a cycle, which means a certain length of time. Now if we talk about cure instead of contagion, it would seem that a certain dose of medicine administered had lasted a certain time.

That is commonly the appearance. The medicine appears to act all that time, and you should be clear in you mind that this is only an appearance. It really means that a certain length of time elapses before another dose is necessary, viz., until another state of susceptibility has arrived. So again we say, whenever a medicine ceases to be homoeopathic it is of no use to administer that medicine any longer, as it will act on the patient only upon an artificial susceptibility. By this we mean that certain sensitive patients always have a susceptibility to high potencies. We have thus two things to deal with, the actuate state, created by the disease itself, and the chronic state, which is the natural state of the patient born under miasm. Now, when in the acute state the patient has satisfied the susceptibility to contagion, there is a period in which the disease cause can no longer operate upon him; he is immune against any further influx of disease cause. But when a remedy ceases to be homoeopathic, the patient has not this immunity against more of its power because of the possibility of variance in the hands of the physician; the potency being given to the patient outside of his own degree of susceptibility, he may be damaged.

---

§ 33. In accordance with this fact it is undeniably shown by all experience that the living human organism is much more disposed and has a greater liability to be acted on and to have its health deranged by medicinal powers, than by morbific noxious agents and infectious miasms; or in other words, *that the morbific noxious agents possess a power of morbidity deranging man's health that is subordinate and conditional, often very conditional; whilst medicinal agents have an absolute unconditional power, greatly superior to the former.*

When we look over the improper use of all sorts of medicines, we can but conclude that the human race, because of drug-taking, has been greatly disordered in the economy. You have heard Hahnemann speak of the management of chronic diseases; he distinctly states that the greatest difficulties are those that have been brought about in the economy by continuous drug taking. It is not that the drugs themselves are laid up in the economy, but that life-long disorder is created. Think of the poor old individuals who were in the habit of taking sulphur and molasses, think of those who were perpetually tapping their livers with blue mass, think of the western sufferers who have filled themselves every year with quinine pan-cake to keep off the chill. These people are so disordered that it takes years of careful prescribing to turn them into a state of order.

In § 34 Hahnemann repeats two propositions to which we have already alluded. The first propositions that in order to cure the medicines must be able to produce in the human body an artificial disease similar to that which is to be cured; this has been fully illustrated and explained. The second proposition is that the artificial disease must be of a greater degree of intensity. The matter of intensity has already been explained as something higher, more internal, something superior or prior. Intensity of power is proportionate to the degree of approximation towards primitive substance. There is no thought of intensity in any other direction. The cause of disease and of cure exists within the primitive substance and not in ultimate material form, although the immaterial cause of disease continues in disease ultimates. The bacteriologists have crawled into confusion because they do not know in their science that causes continue into effects. The bacteria may contain cause because causes are continued into ultimates; but the primitive case is not in the bacteria; the bacteria themselves have a cause.

Classroom Notes

Susceptibility

These paragraphs have a bearing upon the degree or intensity or plane, upon the repetition of dose and upon susceptibility.

These are the things that must be known to become a good prescriber.

[Para: 31]

Disposition and susceptibility are the cause of diseases that allow noxious agents to change health of man and begin disease.

[Para: 32 and 33]

1. Hahnemann states, that we have more power over human beings with drugs than the disease has. A man is only susceptible to natural disease upon a certain plane but we can change potencies of drugs to suit different planes.

2. In cure we have the advantage of change in potency, and this enables us to suit the varying susceptibilities of sick man.

3. Disease causes (which are non-material invisible substances) flow into man's internal state in spite of his protective mechanism and these make him sick. As changes occur in the internal state that bar out any more influx of disease causes then man ceases to be susceptible and there is no longer an inflowing of cause into his economy. A suspension of cause takes place because susceptibility ceases.

Remember disposition is from without and susceptibility is from within.

When does a Homeopathic medicine, administered cease to be Homeopathic?

1. Any amount more than just enough to correct the susceptibility is a surplus and is dangerous.

For example in a chronic disease when it is clearly indicated, Sulphur is administrated and the symptoms disappear and patient feels better then the remedy ceases to be Homeopathic because now it is not required and if administered longer than that, then it becomes surplus hence it is neither homeopathic nor desirable.

2.   Enough medicine must be given to establish order, and that is done almost instantaneously. At the most it is but a matter of a few hours, and as long as order continues after it has once begun keep your hands off.

LECTURE XV

§ 35, ECT. Protection from Sickness

FROM these paragraphs we see that there are several kinds of protection from sickness. When a violent epidemic is raging we all know that, although the number of victims is large, they are few compared to those who go through the epidemic unscathed, and the question always arises, why is it? We suppose, and probably rightly so, that a large number of the immune have escaped because they were usually strong and vigorous, or in a state of very good order. But we find among those who have escaped the epidemic a number of persons who are anything but strong, really invalids, one in consumption, another in the last stages of Bright's disease, another with diabetes. We call them all together and find that none of them have had dysentery or smallpox, or whatever disease was epidemic. They have not been susceptible to epidemic influences. How are you going to explain this? The reason is that they have sickness that it is impossible for the epidemic to suppress. The epidemic is allopathic, or dissimilar to their diseases, and cannot suppress their disease because of its virulency. Now if they have some mild form of chronic disease, a severe attack of dysentery will cause that disease to disappear temporarily, and the new (epidemic) disease will take hold and run its course, and when it subsides the old symptoms will come back again and go on as if they had not been meddled with. This is an illustration of dissimilar, and shows that dissimilars are unable to cure: they can only suppress. If the chronic disease is stronger than the epidemic disease, *i.e.*, if it has an organic hold upon the body, it cannot be suppressed. This is essentially the relation of the acute dissimilar disease to the chronic disease of severity.

The relation between chronic dissimilar diseases is somewhat different. For example, a patient is in the earlier stage of Bright's disease, and the symptoms are clear enough to make a diagnosis. He takes syphilis, and at once the kidney disease is held in abeyance, the albumin disappears from the urine and his waxiness is lost. But after a year's careful prescribing the syphilitic state disappears, and very soon the albumin appears again in the urine, the dropsy returns and he dies of an ordinary attack of Bright's disease.

Then there are cases where two chronic diseases seem at times to alternate with each other; one seems to be subdued for a time and the other prevails. Under proper homoeopathic treatment one will be reduced in its activity and the other chronic disease will show itself. This you will find to be the case when you have to treat syphilis and psora together. The psoric patient, who has been suffering from a skin eruption or one of the various forms of psora, takes syphilis. All the psoric manifestations, the nightly itching of the salt Rheum will disappear, and the syphilitic eruption will come on and take their place. You will treat the syphilitic manifestations for a while and you will be able to subdue them, and in proportion as the disease is subdued the psoric manifestations will come up again and will hold in abeyance that portion of the syphilitic state which is still uncured. You will then be compelled to drop the anti-syphilitic and take up the anti-psoric treatment, and again the homoeopathic remedies will restore apparent order in the economy. But after this has been done, you will be surprised to see syphilitic state return in the condition corresponding to its last manifestations. You must then drop the anti-psoric treatment and resume the anti-syphilitic. Thus they alternate;

when you weaken one, the stronger comes up. The uncomplicated syphilitic eruption does not itch; but the psoric eruption as a rule is an itching eruption, and this will be seen in the alternation of the two diseases.

If the patient is given proper treatment his condition will be simplified, but if given old school treatment it will become very complicated. The two miasms will unite and form a complexity, which is a most vicious state of affairs; then the syphilitic eruptions, while they have all the appearance of syphilis, will itch as if they were psoric eruptions. Mercury in large doses is capable of bringing about such a result. Proper homoeopathic treatment causes a separation, while inappropriate treatment produces complication, and you will never see one improve where homoeopathic remedies have caused the tying up of the combination.

Again, take a chronic malarial diatheses, which has existed so long that it has complicated itself with psora, we will see after the quinine has been antidoted that the chills and fever will come back in their original form. Here you see an evidence of the separation which homeopathy always tends to bring about. The malarial state is now brought into observation for the purpose of cure. It cannot be cured when complicated, for the remedy cannot be clear that will be similar enough to wipe them out. The first prescription antidotes the drug and liberates the patient from the drug disease, and then you see the most acute or last appearing natural disease which comes back first. This is in accordance with fixed law; the last miasm or the last symptoms that have been made to disappear will be the first to return and go away to appear no more.

In § 36 another thought comes up: "Thus non-homoeopathic treatment, which is not violent, leaves the chronic disease unaltered. To suppress, there is required a state of violence to be brought about upon the body; one must do violence to the economy by enormous dosing, tremendous physic, much sweating, blood letting, etc., such as was done in olden times. Such treatment tends to subdue or suppress disease for the time being; but when the violence has subsided and the rough treatment is removed then the symptoms come back, but in a more disturbed state than before. The more violent the drug disease that can be established upon the body the greater the changes in the chronic disease. Violent treatment alers the nature of the chronic diseases. A new and more intense disease suspends a prior dissimilar one existing in the body; similarly, just so long as the effect of quinine continues, so long will it suppress and hold in abeyance the disease to which it is dissimilar. Quinine is capable of engrafting upon the economy its own disease form which will last for years and may not stop until it has been antidoted by a medicine similar to its symptoms. But if it is antidoted, that malarial disease which it suppressed will appear in its original form and the patient will say: "These are just the symptoms I had in the first place when I was cured by the late doctor So-and-so; he cured me with Peruvian bark." That story is so common that any homoeopathic physician who has been doing sound prescribing for years has lots of records of just such cases. The malaria was subdued only because the quinine was capable of producing a more violent disease than malaria. Arsenicum is capable of doing the same thing; it can engraft upon the economy a dangerous disease that will result in very serious conditions because the Arsenicum will complicate itself with psora.

In some cases we have a complexity of horrible things, like one built upon another, and when this is so, in treating them the last group which was removed will appear first, which shows that the remedy has done its work, and we then go on to the next, and so on, the different groups sometimes appeared one after another in distant form. They must disappear in the reverse order of their coming, as if put on in layers, one piled upon another.

From all this we see how it is possible for two different diseases to occupy, as it were, two different corners of the same economy, one manifesting itself while the other is subdued. We also see how they may exist in a state of complexity. In the first instance they do not combine, in the other they do and become complex. We also see the propriety and use of obsreving what treatment has been adminstered to the patient. It is not always possible to do this, and it is impossible to know whether each one of these drugs has established its own disease.

Not every drug that is adminstered is capable of establishing a disease. It is always prudent, when symptoms are only partially developed, and when the drug which caused the suppression of symptoms is known, to include the antidotal relation to the durg with the rest of the systems; that is to say, select a drug which has a well-known antidotal relation to the drug that caused the suppression of the symptoms, providing it is also the most similar of all drugs to the few symptoms that are present. In that way we make as much of similitude as is possible. The similar remedy is most likely of all others to antidote that drug. Do not be led aside to administer right away the drug that caused the trouble. The principle of *Similia* is first.

---

43. Totally different, however, is the result when *two similar* diseases meet together in the organism; that is to say, when to the disease already present a stronger similar one is added. In such cases we see how a cure can be effected by the operations of nature, and we get a lesson as to how man ought to cure.

Then a real conjunction takes place, a union, as it were, a marriage, which results in the disappearance of old things and new things come and exist in a state of order.

Classroom Notes

Protection From Sickness

[Para: 35]

1. From reading this paragraph we see how it is possible for two different diseases to occupy as it were two different corners of the same economy. One manifesting itself while

the order is subdued. They do not combine.

2. In curing such groups, the disease must disappear in the reverse order of their coming, as if, put on in layers, one piled upon the other.

3. Sometimes the two dissimilar diseases combine and become complex. This complex disease presents many difficulties to the physician.

4. When symptoms are masked and when you know the drug, which has caused the masking (suppression of symptom) it is wise to select a drug which has a well known antidotal relation to the drug that cause the suppression of the symptoms. Provided it is also the most similar of all drugs to a few original symptoms that are present.

5. Do not be led aside to administer, right away the drug, that caused the trouble. The principle of similia is first.

[Para: 43]

If two similar diseases meet together in an organism (the natural disease and the artificial disease caused by rightly chosen Homeopathic remedies based on the principle of Similia), then a real conjunction takes place. A union, as it were, which results in disappearance of old things and new state comes and exists in a state of order.

There are two forms of protection from sickness:

(a) Natural Immunity,

(b) Homeopathy.

You will find that for prophylaxis there is required a less degree of similitude than it is necessary for curing. A remedy will not have to be so similar to prevent disease as to cure it.

This is the value and rationale of finding a genus epidemicus after working in an epidemic for few weeks.

LECTURE XVI

§ 44, ETC. Oversensitive Patients

DRUG poisoning such as we referred to in last lecture is not always due to the prescribing of crude drugs. If you work long among sensitive patients you will come across those who have been actually poisoned by the inappropriate administration of potentized medicines. These are oversensitive patients who have received repeated doses of medicine after the medicine and dose that was homoeopathic to their condition was administered.

If a drug that is really homoeopathic to the case is continued, after enough has been given to cure, a miasm is established in some cases by that drug, and this miasm imitates one of the chronic diseases or one of the acute miasms in accordance with its ability. I have a patient who has been suffering for seven or eight years from the effects of Lachesis mutus. I have patients who are suffering from Sulphur and other deep acting medicines which have been repeated too often when truly indicated, or repeated in sensitive patients when not truly indicated. The symptoms of the drug crop out periodically years after it has been abused, and the periodical attacks are perfectly typical of the drug. The mineral substances which are perfectly harmless on the crude plane may be poisonous on the dynamic plane, when the patient is oversensitive. There are persons who can drink a glass of milk with impunity and be nourished by it, but upon whom a drop of milk, potentized to a high degree and repeated beyond its homoeopathicity, will establish a miasm that will last for years. A prover of Lac-canium had a return of its symptoms periodically. She was oversensitive and proved the medicine indiscriminately, and has suffered ever since from its poisonous effect, whereas if it had been given prudently, the disease would have established itself upon the body like any other acute miasm, would have run its course and disappeared. It is unwise to make provings upon oversensitive subjects in that way. I tested a very high potency of Lachesis mutus on an oversensitive patient, giving but a single dose, and that patient ran the course of the Lachesis mutus disease in about two months; the symptoms disappeared and never retuned. While the Lachesis mutus was in progress the patient's chronic symptoms were suppressed, but after it ran its course and disappeared her chronic symptoms came back. This is in accordance with the doctrines. She was oversensitive, and while the dissimilar Lachesis mutus disease was in full blast her chronic disease was suppressed. These are instance when such a patient is truly homoeopathic to remedy, and if that remedy by repeated after enough (I mean in the internal sense) has been given to cure its cases its homoeopathic relation and acting through the general susceptibility creates a miasm upon this extremely sensitive patient. When a patient is hypersensitive you must avoid the use of the c.m. and other very high potencies, which will make your patient sick, and use instead the 30th and 200ths. In cases where the remedy is indicated such potencies will work quite quickly.

---

§ 49. We should have been able to meet with many more real natural homoeopathic cures of this kind, if, on the one hand, the attention of observers had been more directed to them and, on the other had, if nature had not been so deficient in helpful homoeopathic diseases.

Hahnemann, in § 46, gives examples of these natural cures. We occasionally meet with these cures now. We find patients that are threatened with phthisis go to the South, because it has been proved that such cases can go into a vitiated climate and stay for a number of years, and actually receive benefit from this disease-producing neighbourhood, and go away well. Others go into a climate more wholesome and they are not cured. The miasms can cure all similar diseases, and the curing substances are in attenuated form. The evils that arise from these swamps are similar to the evils of the economy of the patient, and that similitude is antidotal, is curative, and causes change back into order in accordance with the eternal law that governs the action of similars.

There was a time in the early days of homoeopathy when, taking into view the great array of disease forms to be contended with and the very few medicines then at his command, the homoeopath was worried to find remedies similar to all of his cases. That cannot be true now. If the homoeopath will work in a systematic way, he will be able to command enough of the Materia Medica to meet all the diseases that he comes in contact with, the symptoms of which are sufficiently observed.

Every man should put himself to the task of studying the Materia Medica; he has no time to lose, no time to fool away. The physician can really have no excuse at the present day to leave our proved medicines, the medicines that are recorded in our books; he can have no reasonable excuse for stepping aside into ways that are dark, treacherous and recommended only by tradition. Some physicians hold that it is liberal to do anything for a patient. This is a pitfall, a rock, that will destroy any physician that will not avoid it. We know that there are doctors, who claim to be homoeopaths, who attempt or justify, upon some ground or other, the administration of remedies merely to palliate and relieve suffering. With such men there must be a lack of sturdiness in listening of the sufferings of a patient. It seems to me that no one who is honest, and who has knowledge of the stupidity that comes after the administration of a medicine that will cause the symptoms to disappear, will actually tie his hands against the finding of a remedy that will be suitable to cure. As surely as the voice of the symptoms is hushed, so surely does the physician put out of his way the opportunity for selecting a homoeopathic remedy. When the index to the remedy is spoiled the ability of the physician to benefit his patient is destroyed. If you give quinine, go on with it; if you given an opiate, go on with it; do not go back into homoeopathy. This man who does these things is a homoeopathic failure. Some men are incapable of grasping the homoeopathic doctrines, and fall into mongrelism, which is a cross between homoeopathy and allopathy. I would prefer an allopath to one who professes to be a homoeopath, but does not know enough homoeopathy to practice it.

Why should you put crude medicines upon the diphtheritic membrane in addition to giving your remedy? If the crude drugs do anything they will spoil the appearance of the throat, and you will not be able to know what your remedy has done. If these adjuvants to the remedy do anything at all they will effect such changes, as will damage the case; they do not effect changes, why use them? There can be no reason for administering something that does not effect changes. This question came up one time, and created controversy in an association meeting. One doctor recommended the use of Peroxide of Hydrogen in pus cavities; he said it did no harm, it did no damage. The question is, does it do anything at all? If it does, the changes it effects injure the case.

Lay it down, as a rule, that you will use nothing that can effect changes in a case in addition to your remedy. After you prescribe a remedy you want to know when you come back whether that remedy has done anything. For this reason you must rest your case upon that which you believe to be the nearest homoeopathic remedy. All changes must be watched, because by observing changes we know what next to do. If something has been given by the patient's friends and changes have occurred in the case from such meddling the doctor is in confusion. If absolutely no changes have occurred after his remedy then he is in intelligence and knows what next to do.

Doctors sometimes give opium to suppress pain, but it is more frequently given to suppress the cry of people that stand around listening to the patient. The friends stand there wringing their hands and saying: "Doctor, cannot you do something?" and the poor doctor loses his head and gives a dose of opium. What does he do that for? In order to quiet the cry of the people. He knows he is damaging his patient, he knows he has put out off his hands the ability to cure that patient homeopathically. What if the patient does suffer? Can that be an excuse for the doctor destroying his power to heal that patient hereafter? The doctor justifies himself by saying, "If I had not done this the people would have criticized me." What business is it of the people? If a doctor has not the grit to withstand the cries of the family, the criticisms of the friends, the threatening of his pocketbook and of his bread and butter, he will not practice homoeopathy very long. An honest man does not fear these things. There is but one thing for him to consider, what is the right thing he must do. The harangue of the crazy old women who stand around wagging their tattling tongues, what has that to do with the life of patient or the duty of the patient or the duty of the physician? Will they shoulder the responsibility of the patient's death, if he die? I say now that the death of a patient is nothing in comparison with violation of the law on the part of the doctor. In both instances the doctor gets the worst of it. The doctor who violates the law also violates his conscience, and his death is worse than the death of the patient. Generally the physician who has knowledge enough and grit enough to wait will see, before the patient dies, the homoeopathic remedy that will control the case. The whole community is sometimes turned into excitement because a doctor will not do this or that. Suppose the whole atmosphere is blue with effects of their wrath, what has that to do with it? The physician who will stick by the patient and let the people howl is one that will be trusted through any and every ordeal. But the doctor that will flinch and tremble at every threatening is one that will violate his conscience, is one that can be bought, can be hired to do anything, and will abandon his color in time of emergency. It is hard work for a homoeopathic physician to settle off alone by himself where he has nobody that will stand by him in his tribulations. The attitude of the public must never furnish the physician with indications as to what he shall do. Let him study the patient and the symptoms of the patient. That which is right is protected and supported, and that which is wrong degrades. Let a man lose his self-respect a few times and he becomes a coward and a sneak, and is ready to do almost anything that is vicious and cowardly. The physician who has done rightly by his patient can look the friends squarely in the face when the patient has died. If he has administered morphine to the patient and turned aside all the symptoms upon which he could find that remedy, it does not seem to me that he can look the friends squarely in the face. Of course, if you act according to principle in this way you suffer for it. You will be called names.

In the 63rd and 64th paragraphs Hahnemann treats of the primary and secondary actions of medicines. There is no necessity for dwelling upon this subject. The primary and secondary actions of a drug are simply the one action of that drug. Some homoeopaths have attempted to individualize between the primary and secondary action. It does not matter what the patient is suffering from, from symptoms which appeared in the primary action or from symptoms which appeared in the secondary action, that drug will cure just the same. The symptoms that arise are the symptoms that arise from the remedy, and they often seem to oppose each other. In the earlier stages we have sometimes sleeplessness; in the last stages, sleepiness, and one state is sometimes more prominent than the other. For instance in Opium, some provers had sleeplessness first and sleepiness afterwards, from the smaller doses of Opium. It is known that Opium has both sleeplessness and sleepiness, and if the other symptoms agree it does not matter which one of the two is present. If Opium is indicated by the general state of the patient it will cure either of these conditions, and you need not stop to see if it produces one state in one place and the opposite in another. In some provers Opium produces diarrhoea in the beginning, in others constipation. If I should take today a crude does of Opium, in six hours I would have a diarrhoea that would last for several days and then be constipated for six weeks. To know that drugs have two actions is simply knowing the nature of drugs in general. You will find another example in alcohol; watch two drunkards and you will see the double action illustrated.

There are constitutional states in patients by virtue of which they are always affected in a certain way, and these states are often left after provings, or are found in those who have been poisoned by a drug. All these patients will have alternating symptoms which will confuse the physician before he knows their constitutional state. It is an important thing to know the constitutional state of patient before prescribing. You will always be able to do better for your patients when you know all of their tendencies. Of course, in acute diseases symptoms sometimes stand out so sharply that an acute remedy can be administered without reference to any constitutional state. Acute cognates can be established in almost any patient. For instance, the Calcarea carbonica patient will need an acute cognate of Calcarea carbonica when he is sick with acute symptoms. The acute symptoms fits into and are established and formed by the constitutional state of the patient.

Classroom Notes

Oversensitive Patient

[Para: 44]

1. There are constitutional states in patients by virtue of which patients are always affected in a certain way.
2. It is important to know the constitutional state of a patient before prescribing. You will always do better when you know your patients tendencies.
3. Of course in acute diseases symptoms stand out so sharply that acute remedy may be administered without reference to a constitutional state.
4. If the drug is really Homeopathic and is continued even after enough has been given to cure, a miasma is established

in some cases by that drug. This miasma imitates one of the chronic or acute miasma in accordance with its ability.

A mineral substance that is perfectly harmless on a crude plane may be poisonous on the dynamic plane, if the patient is over-sensitive.

When can a Homeopathic remedy harm?

1. Deep acting remedies that have been repeated too often when truly indicated.
2. Deep acting remedies that are given to oversensitive patient when not truly indicated.

When a patient is oversensitive you must avoid the use of the CM and other high potencies, which will make your patient sick. Use instead 30C or the 200c potency.

[Para: 49]

Lay down as a rule, that you will use nothing that can effect changes in a case other than your Homeopathic remedy.

After you have prescribed the medicine you would want to know whether this remedy has done anything. For this reason you must rest your case on that medicine that you believe is the near-est Homeopathic remedy.

All changes must be watched, because by observing changes we know what next to do.

[Para: 63, 64]

Here Hahnemann talks about the primary and secondary action of medicines. There is no necessity for dwelling upon this subject.

LECTURE XVII

The Science and the Art

UP to this time we have been studying principles that relate to the knowledge of homoeopathy. At this point Hahnemann arrives at three important conclusions as to what we have been studying in application to practice. There are three steps to be surveyed :

1st. " By what means is the physician to arrive at the necessary information relative to a disease, in order to be able to undertake the cure"? Of course that relates to the disease in general, and the patient in particular. In going over the 3rd paragraph, we gathered together the means of studying an epidemic and each man in particular. We shall now proceed to study disease in general and the patient in particular, from now on to the end of the course. All the rest of the study is of such a character. There are a great many questions that arise in this problem that must be studied in detail, the study of the nature of acute miasms and the study of the nature of the chronic miasms; the study of such changes as show there are two distinct classes of sickness. Each one is to be studied in its most general way, and each person as a particular entity.

2nd. "How is he to discover the morbific powers of medicines; that is to say, of the instruments destined to cure natural diseases?" This constitutes a study of Materia Medica and a knowledge of how it is built,which is by provings, by recorded facts.

3rd. "What is the best mode of applying these morbific powers (medicines) in the cure of diseases?" This involves the study of all methods and setting upon that which is best.

To proceed in the study of these in a rational, scientific and careful manner is the object of the future study of this book. It leads , from now on , from the science of homoeopathy to the art of healing. We see that we have now gone over the principle part of which is merely science, the science of homoeopathy. We have none of the enormous classifications in the study of homoeopathy that are resorted to in traditional medicine; they should not appear in the study of applied homoeopathy. The study of the classification of disease as is done in traditional medicine is useful, because we come in contact with the world. As the Boards of Health require us to state what particular disease, according to classification , a patient died from, classified in accordance with old school nosology, we have therefore, to go into the study of diagnosis. In homoeopathy, diagnosis cuts very little figure in the treatment; but all the ultimates in the case must be brought forward and described by name. We want the use of adjectives, we want the use of large language, we want descriptive power, in order that nature of sickness, which is all that man can know about the disease, may be brought out on the paper, and thereby caused to appear at any time thereafter to the mind of the physician. If the physician were simply to make a study of the disease, and after studying it were to give it a name and let that name constitute the record, no future prescription could be made. And the physician, thereafter, in referring to this record, would know nothing about its nature. The name conveys no idea of the nature of the sickness, only its place in in a general classification. A knowledge of the nature of individual sickness is necessary for a prescription , and this depends upon the ascertainment of the details.

The very first of this study is to prove and realize that there are two classes of diseases, acute and chronic. The general classification of all diseases is made in this way; the acute are thrown into one group and studied as acute diseases, and so with the chronic.

An acute miasm is one that comes upon the economy passes

through its regular prodromal period, longer or shorter, has its period of progress and the period of decline, and in which there is a tendency to recovery. A chronic miasms is one that has its period of prodrome, period of progress and no period of decline; it is continuous, never ending, except with the death of the patient.

The acute diseases need much less study than the chronic. They are all such as are contagious or infectious, such as have a miasmatic character and are capable of running a definite course. When man disorders his stomach and has an attack of vomiting, and from which he has no after trouble, he has suffered merely from an indisposition. Such conditions from external causes are not miasms. Things that go through the mouth into the stomach and thereby produce sickness act either as rousers up of the some old trouble or as mechanical causes of disturbance. The pure disease, on the other hand, whether acquired or inherited , are those that flow from the innermost to the outermost while making man sick. These causes that make man sick are influx of simple substance and they run in a fixed distinct course. Each one has its own time of prodrome, its own period of progress, whereby the traditional school of medicine has fixed what it calls pathognomonic symptoms. It is well to know these symptoms, not for the purpose of naming merely, but for the purpose of association.

The study of disease should not be for the purpose of naming; if it is so, the name does harm. When you think of a child suffering from measles, the idea of measles may go out of mind, but the character of the sickness of that particular child must remain in the mind. At first you will not be able to see what is meant by that, especially if you have been in the habit of studying cases for the purpose of diagnosis.

I do not say this to throw a cloud upon diagnosis, but to show that the study of diagnosis is not for the purpose of making a prescription. The more you swell upon diagnostics symptoms, the more you will becloud the ideas entering the mind that lead toward a prescription. You might go into the room and work an hour individualizing a case, deciding whether it were measles or scarlet fever (there are some confusing cases in the beginning).

Well, you might say, it is measles, and must now have Pulsatilla nigricans, or scarlet fever and must have Belladonna. You will really see that such a state of affairs is misleading to the mind. If you are in an epidemic, where it is necessary in order to save the neighbourhood, to know, for instance, whether a certain case is of cholera or not, then it becomes necessary to do the two things. The family and the surrounding families are entitled to the safety that a correct knowledge would give and that protection, isolation or quarantine would afford. There are two kinds of study, one with a bearing toward the classification that the disease belongs to, and one with reference to the remedy that the patient needs; but I pre- fer to settle the patient first as to the remedy he needs, and this has very little to do with the classification, except in a general way. After a remedy has been decided upon that clearly covers the symptoms and the patient receives his dose of medicine, the next point is, what step is necessary to take in order to protect the peo- ple if this is a contagious disease. Diagnosis is something that a physician cannot afford to go around calling scarlet fever measles, and measles scarlet fever. He must know enough about the gener- al nature of diseases that after the prescription has been made and the patient settled as to that, and the mother wants to know what is the matter with the child, to tell her, for, in that instance, she has a perfect right to know; that is, a case where the family must be protected, where outsiders must be protected; the physician must decide whether it is proper for the child to go to school, or whether it is not proper.

There are some conditions of chronic diseases which closely resemble acute diseases; for instance, these mimicking acute attacks that come on regularly as periodical headaches. One attack, singled out, might have the appearance of an acute miasm, yet the tendency to progress and not to recovery shows that it belongs to the chronic class. Those disorders that come from debauchery and drinking and overeating, from immediate circum- stances that are periodical, are things that arise from the latent psoric condition; they are momentary sickness, and if it were not for the fact that man suffers from chronic miasms he would not have these; these attacks would not form a sickness, would not have an appearance of acute sickness. It is due to chronic miasms that man has these little recurring attacks. These do not come with a prodromal period, a progressive period and a period of decline; they may have an attack and decline, but not a prodrome. The acute miasms like the chronic have the prodromal period.

Par. 72 says: "Relative to the first point, it will be necessary for us to enter here into some general considerations. The diseases of man resolve themselves into two classes," etc. Remember that the acute diseases always tend to recovery; the chronic diseases have no tendency whatever to recovery, but a continuous progressive tendency; they are far deeper miasms.

There are three of these chronic miasms that belong to the human family - psora, syphilis and sycosis - and these we will take up and study. The worst cases are those wherein the three chronic miasms, or some parts of the three, have been complicated by drugs. When the effect of drugs has been removed then we may begin to study the pure miasms themselves, but the miasms are complicated at the present day in most men, for whenever we come in contact with chronic sickness we come in contact also with chronic drugging and its effect upon the vital force. I am of the opinion, perhaps I am wrong, that when blood-letting was in vogue, when violent cathartics were thrown in, when emetics and sweating were prescribed, as in the olden times, when all these violent things were resorted to, the human race was not torn to pieces as rapidly as at the present day. The enormous doses of Jalap and Calomel rushed through the intestines and cleaned out the patient, and he felt better afterwards, and probably did not carry to his grave the internal results of that cleaning out. He did not carry the internal results of the emetics and sudorifics, but at the present day small doses of concentrated drugs are administered, which have an insidious effect upon the economy and develop their chronic symptoms very slowly. From the continued taking of old school products, the alkaloids, etc., we have the most dreadful state that has ever occurred in the history of medicine coming on. The aim is to get small doses, to get an insidious effect. The milder preparations, like Sulphonal, require months to develop their chronic tendencies, and are most vicious and troublesome drugs. These slow and subtle preparations are now being manufactured, and though seeming to produce a mild primary effect have secondary effects or after effects which are very severe. Hahnemann said, in his time, the most troublesome chronic diseases were those that had been complicated with drugs. If that were true then it is ten times so now. The little headache compounds, the catarrh cures, etc., are milder as to the first effects, but more violent as to the last effects. They are prepared to imitate the palatable form of homoeopathic remedies.

Classroom Notes

Homeopathy: Science and Art

Up to this time we have studied the principle that relate to the knowledge of Homeopathy. At this point, Hahnemann arrives at three important conclusions as to what we have to study with application, to practice.

These are:

1. By what means the physician shall arrive at the necessary information related to a disease. In order to undertake a cure. This constitutes, what is curable in a disease.

2. The study of Materia Medica and a knowledge how it is built i.e. drug proving. This constitutes, what is curative in a medicine.

3. What is the best mode of applying these artificial morbific powers (medicines) to cure a disease, i.e. how to adapt?

To proceed in the study of these three objectives, in a reason oriented scientific manner, is the aim of further study of this book.

We shall proceed to study disease in general and the patient in particular from now up to the end of this book.

Knowledge of nature of individual sickness is necessary for prescription and this depends upon study of symptoms prior to the pathology.

The more you dwell upon diagnostic symptoms, the more you will be clear regarding the ideas entering one's mind that lead towards a prescription.

There are two kinds of thoughts/ study:

1. Study of symptoms, with a bearing towards the diagnostic classification to which the disease belongs.

2. The study of symptoms with reference to what remedy the patient needs.

Kent's formula of management of disease.

"I prefer to settle the patient first to what remedy he needs and this has very little to do with diagnostic classification expect in a general way. After the remedy is decided upon I decide upon the dose [amount and potency] that the patient receives.

After a remedy has been decided upon that clearly covers the symptoms and the patient has received his dose of medicine.

The next point is what steps are necessary in order to protect the patient if it is a non-contagious disease and to protect other people if it is a contagious disease."

LECTURE XVIII

Chronic Diseases—Psora

PSORA is the beginning of all physical sickness. Had psora never been established as a miasm upon the human race, the other two chronic diseases would have been impossible, and susceptibility to acute diseases would have been impossible. All the disease of man are built upon psora; hence it is the foundation of sickness; all other sickness came afterwards.

Psora is the underlying cause, and is the primitive or primary disorder of the human race. It is a disordered state of the internal economy of the human race. This state expresses itself in the forms of the varying chronic diseases, or chronic manifestations. If the human race had remained in a state of perfect order, psora could not have existed. The susceptibility to psora opens out a question altogether too broad to study among the sciences in a medical college. It is altogether too extensive, for it goes to the very primitive wrong of the human race, the very first sickness of the human race, that is the spiritual sickness, from which first state the race progressed into what may be called the true susceptibility to psora, which in turn laid the foundation for other diseases. If we regard psora as synonymous with itch, we fail to understand, and fail to express thereby, anything like the original intention of Hahnemann. The itch is commonly supposed to be a limited thing, something superficial, caused by a little tiny but of a mite that is supposed to have life, and when the little itch mite is destroyed the cause of itch is said to have been removed. What a folly!

From a small beginning with wonderful progress, psora spreads out into its underlying states and manifests itself in the large portion of the chronic diseases upon the human race. It embraces epilepsy, insanity, the malignant diseases, tumors, ulcers, catarrhs, and a great proportion of the eruptions. It progresses from simple states to the very highest degree of complexity, not always alone and by itself, but often by the villainous aid of drugging during generation after generation; for the physician has endeavored with all his power to drive it from the surface, and has thereby caused it to root itself deeper, to become more dense and invisible, until the human race is almost threatened with extinction. Look at the number of the population upon the face of the earth, and notice how few arrive at the age of maturity. It is appalling to think of the number of infants that die, and these largely from the outgrowths, or outcoming of psora. We see little ones born who have not sufficient vitality to live. The congenital debility, and marasmus, and varying diseases of a chronic character that carry off the little ones have for their underlying cause the chronic miasms. The principal underlying cause is psora, next syphilis and next sycosis.

It required twelve years for Hahnemann to discover and gather together the evidence upon which he came to his conclusions. When a patient came to him who manifested chronic disease in any way he took pains to write down carefully in detail all the symptoms, from beginning to end, with the history of the father and mother, until he had collected a great number of appearances of disease, not knowing yet what the outcome would be; but after this careful writing out of the symptoms of hundreds of patients, little and great, and comparing them and then gathering them together in one grand group, there appeared in the totality of this collection a picture of psora in all its forms. Up to this time the world has been looking upon each one of these varying forms as distinct in itself, *e.g.,* all the striking features of epilepsy would be gathered together, and epilepsy was then called a disease; but epilepsy is only one of the results of disease, and never appears twice alike. Every person who has epilepsy differs from every other epileptic on earth. But epilepsy, insanity, diabetes, cancer Bright's disease, and every other case of so-called disease have all had a beginning and one beginning. They are not distinct, but operate in each person in accordance with that individual. Hahnemann says that before he began that collection of symptoms he was struck somewhat with wonder that Nux vomica and Ignatia amara and such short acting medicines were able to cure only a single manifestation of disease, a group of symptoms, or they would relieve for a time and then the symptoms would come back, although he had followed up the treatment to the best of his knowledge. At the end of a case, he could discover that there had been a continuous progress in spite of the fact that he had relieved his patient of suffering a good many times.

So it is, while acute acting remedies are used, and you will use them if you do not know the psoric doctine. The short acting medicines are the ones that contain the counterparts of the acute manifestations of psora, and hence when these acute manifestations appears in groups of symptoms you will naturally select acute remedies, and you will palliate them from time to time, but at the end of years you will look upon every individual case, and will notice that the case has been steadily progressing. You will find that you have not struck at the root of the trouble, that there is an underlying something present and prevailing and that the disease is steadily growing worse.

Hahnemann saw this and it was a mystery to him because he had acquired a perfect mastery over the acute disease with the acute remedies. Such apsorics had been at this time very well proved, Belladonna, Aconitum napellus, Bryonia alba, Arnica montana, China, Nux vomica, etc., etc., and these had been found to be perfectly suitable for the acute manifestations of psora and for the acute miasms. Hahenemann had not yet learned that the acute miasms were utterly and strictly acute miasms; and could not, therefore, compare acute miasms with chronic miasms, or vice versa. He had not seen them yet as miasms.

One will not understand the acute miasms clearly until able to compare them with chronic miasms. They side up one with another, and make it wonderfully manifest. The acute miasms come on either with sufficient violence to cause death to patients, or with less violence, wherein there is a period of progress and a tendency to recover. They cannot be prolonged in the patient, and must subside. The acute miasms are not governed in accordance with fixed time in order to be acute miasms, because they have time of their own. Neither is there a time after the lapse of which the chronic miasms is said to be chronic. According to the old school, diseases have been divided into acute, sub-acute and chronic. If any sickness ran longer than six weeks, it would be place among the sub-acute; if it ran on indefinitely, it was called chronic. But a chronic miams is chronic from its beginning, and an acute miasm is acute from its beginning. It is from its nature, from its capabilities, from what it will do to the human race, that we must name the miasm.

So Hahenemann tells us frankly that he was astonished to find at the end of a certain length of time no progress had been made with his remedies in chronic diseases. The symptoms appeared with their own regularity, much stronger than before, which showed they were progressing. Hahenemann enters not only a difficult study, but with all sorts of difficulties, and after studying for twelve years he developed the fact that in all cases observed there was an underlying chronic disease, a chronic miasm, which had a tendency to progress and to end only with the life of the patient. Then he bent himself to the provings of medicines in order to discover from them a likeness to the chronic miasms. Had he never come to this conclusion, he would not have noticed such things.

When he had bought all the symptoms before the mind in one grand collective view, he began to observe and reflect as to what was the first, and what was the second, and later appearances in the line of progress in this deep-seated chronic miasm. Thus it was that he observed amongst those who were dying with phthisis that in their younger days they had a vesicular disease between the fingers and upon the body, which had been suppressed by the ointments in vogue at that time. Then the question naturally arose, what had this suppression to do with that which came afterwards? As to how Hahnemann figured out the answer to that question you can read in his "Chronic Diseases," but he does not tell it all; although he gives many pages of experiences and observations. You will more clearly understand and be better prepared to take up Hahnemann's line of thinking, if you enter into the use of appropriate medicines and apply principle to the progress of disease-that is, you will see a demonstration of his teaching in the curative treatment of a very large number of cases of sickness by applying principles: that diseases get will in the reverse order in which they appeared; old symptoms, in the form of eruptions, come back, old chills, which have been suppressed, come back, and many other chronic manifestations come back again in a sort of successive order. If we observed these things we must come to the conclusion that when we have driven these oldest and deepest troubles back to their original manifestations, which was perhaps a vesicular eruption, and if we see nothing more simple than this eruption, we must conclude that the suppression of such an eruption was the beginning of trouble.

If you practice accurately, you will observe these things; if you are not a success in practice, you will not observe these things. Many patients are so badly off that this is never observed, and then we have the onward progress; that is, we have the patient declining, instead of the disease declining. If that patient is only better as to symptoms, and his old symptoms do not come back, we know that he is only being palliated, that the disease processes are only being restrained, but that it is not a case of cure. There is one thing that you should know and it is sometimes best to say it to the patient, and that is that they should not take too much courage, because a patient that takes too much courage may take too much discouragement when reverses come. So when a woman walks into your office and says beautiful things by way of gratitude for what you have done for her, because you have mitigated the deep-seated trouble, perhaps chronic sick headache, or epilepsy, but she cannot tell you of an eruption returning or you have observed no backward progress of that disease, no reverse order of the symptoms, it is often well to say to that patient, that not-withstanding the fact that she appears to be much improved the trouble is not over for all that. On the other hand, it is sometimes wise to say: "If an eruption should come out, do not on your life meddle with it," because they will probably use what they say relieved it in the first place, some Sulphur ointment, or some other miserable stuff. The physician should bear in mind to caution the patient against removing any of the symptoms in the case. When the patient comes and reports such wonderful tales of progress, take down your record and look it over. If you have in the record failed to get the earlier history of the case, endeavour then, if possible, to find out something about the previous symptoms, the earlier symptoms, and then it is sometimes well with an intelligent person to say: "Do not be surprised, do not be alarmed, if such and such symptoms return," cautioning the patient to report to the physician and apply nothing. Now, it is from these circumstances that we observe finally, where the patient is so well instructed not to do anything, to take no drugs, to keep the life as pure as possible, to keep the physical forces untrammeled by violence, it is under such circumstances that we shall observe the coming back of symptoms that have long been suppressed. Long after the treatment has ceased, a patient will come back and say: "This old trouble has come back on me; can you do anything for it?" You have now to look over the record, and you see that sure enough this is like what came out in the beginning of this trouble; that psora existed in its simplest form of a vesicular eruption upon the child, and that it was suppressed.

These are the simplest cases of psora, because these can be counted collectively in one person; but the complicated forms of psora are those that are inherited. Amongst the simple forms of psora, after the eruptions disappear, catarrhal troubles come on, with their varying manifestations. You prescribe for all these symptoms, and presently the eruptions of childhood come back, especially in a younger person. If it is in a more complicated state, we do not get the patient back to the original form of psora, because the parent had the simple form of psora, and the child gets a complex form from those which were present when the patient came to you. You will seldom see the vesicular form or simple form brought back except in those who have had the simple form, but forms approximating the simple will return if the vital energy of the economy is being turned into order.

Since this, then, is the natural form of economy, we see we are gradually travelling back towards the beginning of psora or its earlier forms. If you are treating a vicious form of scaly eruptions, dry hard horney scales, you will, under accurate prescribing, notice these scaly formations disappear, but after the vital force has become strong enough you need not be surprised to see *vesicular* eruptions develop, for the original so-called disease had changed from its vicious squamos form to the milder vesicular form. Different names have been given to the skin diseases, but we see that names are of very little value. The different eruptions change into varying forms but they are all from one cause, and will come back in their successive stages under true homoeopathic treatment. This is seen quite often enough to demonstrate what I am talking about, and from this alone we can ascertain that psora begins with the simple isolated vesicular form of eruption. At times you will be treating the more advanced and complicated forms of psora, where there are organic changes; after the patient gets the homoeopathic remedy for a while he comes to a standstill, seems to be doing nothing, but in the course of time vicious ugly eruptions came out upon the body. This is a good sign in so far as the disease manifests itself upon the skin, or in catarrhal discharges, the internal organs are safe, but when these outward manifestations are stopped the internal parts suffer.

If this be true, what conclusion must we come to as to the good or injury done to patients when every catarrhal discharge is stopped and every eruption upon the skin is driven away by outward applications? What are we to conclude when we see that the idea of the medical world of today is to stop everything-that appears upon the surface? When we know the truth in regard to psora, we see what a wonderful damage it is to the patient to have these outward signs stopped in this way, what a tremendous shock it is to the economy, and how it is that psora is pushed on and made worse, made more complex from year to year, from generation to generation, until it is the fundamental disease of the human economy and the basis of all the trouble in man.

At the present day, as you are now prepared to hear, we can really learn more about psora by watching it in its backward progress than by watching it in its onward progress in any particular case. It is the cause of the chronic manifestations of disease that are not syphilitic or sycotic. We are able to group together in the mind all those vicious constitutional states (not syphilitic or sycotic) that are called organic disease, as the results of psora. Then the five forms of Bright's disease are not diseases, but the result of psora operating upon the economy and attacking the kidney. The common chronic diseases of the liver are not diseases, but the localization of psora in the liver; the lung diseases and heart diseases and brain diseases are not diseases, because they have one single origin, and from this origin we follow their progress and thus study them from their beginnings to their ends, from cause to ultimates. Only in this way will we have a clear knowledge of their internal cause and beginnings.

Classroom Notes

Chronic Disease—Psora

Psora is the beginning of all physical sickness.

1.   Had Psora never been established as a miasma upon the human race, the other chronic diseases (sycosis, syphilis, tuberculosis, cancer.) would have been impossible, and susceptibility to acute diseases would also have been impossible. All the diseases of mankind are built upon Psora. Hence it is the foundation of all sickness.

2.   **Psora** is the underlying cause, and it is the primitive or primary disorder of the human race. It is the disordered state of the internal economy of the human race. This state expresses

itself in the form of various chronic manifestations, the so called chronic diseases.

3. The study of susceptibility to Psora, is altogether too extensive, for it goes to the very primitive wrong of the human race. Psora is spiritual sickness (*by spiritual sickness Kent means a sickness of the spirit that is to say the sickness of the realm of thought and emotion*).

4. From this first state, the human race has progressed into what may be called the true susceptibility to Psora, which in turn has laid the foundation for other diseases.

5. If we regard Psora as synonymous with itch, we fail to understand, and fail to express thereby the original intention of Hahnemann. It embraces diseases like: epilepsy, insanity, the malignant diseases, tumors, ulcers, catarrhs, and a great proportion of the eruptions. From beginning minute Psora progresses into its underlying states and manifests itself in the large proportion of the chronic disease of high degree of complexity.

6. To understand Hahnemann's intention we must perceive why he thought of miasma or such a thing anyway. It may be mentioned here that Hahnemann took twelve years to gather evidence, upon which he came to this conclusions.

7. Types of Diseases:
    According to the school of the day, diseases were divided into: acute, sub-acute and chronic.
    (a) The acute diseases were those diseases that came on either with sufficient violence to cause death of patients. Or with less violence, where there was a period of progress and a tendency to recover.
    (b) If any sickness ran longer than six weeks, it would be placed among the sub-acute.
    (c) If it ran on indefinitely, it was called as chronic.

8. Hahnemann saw in his practice that his patients recovered from acute diseases quite rapidly but they came back with the same or some other disease and it was a mystery to him because he thought he had acquired a mastery over the acute diseases with his apsorics (acute remedies). Such apsorics like

Belladonna, Aconite, Bryonica, Arnica, China, Nux Vomica, etc, had been by this time very well proved by him.

9. Concept of Chronic Diseases—

    Hahnemann soon realized that a chronic miasma is indefinite from its very beginning, and an acute miasma is short - acting from its start. It is from its nature, from its capabilities and from what it will do to the human race, that we must name the miasma.

10. This thought dawned only when he had brought all the symptoms before his mind, in one grand collective view. He began to observe and reflect as to which symptoms were the first, and which the second were, and other later appearances in the line of progress of this deep-seated chronic miasma. Thus it was observed by Hahnemann that among those who were dying with phthisis, in their younger days they had a vesicular disease between the fingers and upon the body, which had been suppressed by the ointments in vogue at that time. Then the question naturally arise—

    • What had this suppression to do with the disease that came afterwards?

    • As to how Hahnemann figured out the answer to that question one can read in his "Chronic Diseases".

11. One can clearly understand and better prepared to take up Hahnemann's line of thinking, if one will see a demonstration of his teaching in the curative treatment of a very large number of cases of sickness by applying his principles of cure.

12. Diseases get well in the reverse order of their coming. That is the latest symptoms will be the first to go away, and that the older symptoms will at last, that is in reverse order in which they appeared, e.g.:

    • Old symptoms, in the form of eruptions, came back.

    • Old chills, which have been suppressed, came back.

    • Many other chronic manifestations came back again in a sort of successive order.

13. If we observe these things we come to the conclusion that when we have driven these oldest and deepest troubles back to perhaps a vesicular eruption, we must conclude that the sup-

pression of such a eruption has been the beginning of trouble.

14. If one practices accurately, one will observe these things. If one is not a success in practice, he or she will not observe these things. Always tell the patient, "do not be surprised, do not be alarmed, if such and such symptoms return". Caution the patient to report to the physician and do nothing by himself, to alter such a response. These above mentioned are simplest cases of Psora, because these can be observed collectively in one person.

Inherited Psora

15. The complicated forms of Psora are those that are inherited. If one is treating a vicious form of scaly eruption; dry, hard, horny scales. Under accurate prescribing, one will notice these scaly formations disappear, but after the vital force has become strong enough one need not be surprised to see vesicular eruptions develop, because the original so-called disease has changed from its vicious squamous from to the milder vesicular form. This is good sign as far as the disease manifests itself upon the skin, or in catarrhal discharges. The internal organs are safe, but when these outward manifestations are stopped, the internal parts suffer.

16. We can really learn more about Psora by watching it, in its backward progression than by watching it, in its forward progression in any particular case. We are able to group together in the mind all those vicious constitutional states (not Syphilitic or Sycotic) that are called organic disease, as the result of Psora.

17. According to Hahnemann, the five forms of Bright's disease, chronic diseases of liver, lungs, heart, brain and other such organs are result of Psora operating from within. They are not individual disease entities, but it is Psora operating in each sick person in accordance to the susceptibility of that individual. From this origin we as Homeopaths, follow the disease; from it's begining to it's end and from cause to ultimates. Only in this way we will have a a clear knolwedge of the internal cuase and begining of miasmatic disease.

LECTURE XIX

Chronic Diseases—Psora *(Continued)*

IN the work on "Chronic diseases" Hahnemann refers to psora as the oldest, most universal and most pernicious chronic miasmatic disease, yet it has been misappropriated more than any other. "Psora is the oldest miasmatic chronic disease known. The oldest history of the oldest nation does not reach its origin. Psora is just as tedious as syphilis and sycosis, and is, moreover, hydra-headed. Unless it is thoroughly cured, it lasts until the last breath of the longest life. Not even the most robust constitution by its own unaided efforts, is able to anninilate and extinguish psora".

The three chronic miasms, psora, syphilis and sycosis, are all contagious. In each instance there is something prior to the manifestations which we call disease. We speak of the signs and symptoms of a disease, we speak of the outcroppings of the symptoms when we speak of syphilis , but remember there is a state prior to syphilis or syphilis would not exist. It could not come upon man except for a condition suitable to its development. In like manner psora could not exist except for a condition in mankind suitable for its development.

Psora being the first and the other two coming later, it is proper for us to inquire into that state of the human race that would be suitable for the development of psora. There must have been a state of the human race suitable to the development of psora; it could not have come upon a perfectly healthy race, and it would not exist in a perfectly healthy race. There must have been some sickness prior to this state, which we recognize as the chronic miasm psora; some state of disorder, some state that it would be perfectly rational and proper for man to undertake to solve as to its cause, as to its history, and as to its very nature. Some will say, but if we undertake to do this we will have to accept the word of God as historical, as relating to the beginning, because there is no other going so far back. There is no harm in reasoning from that and I hope you will so accept it, not only as history, but as divine revelation, not that I wish to quote from or refer to it, because I never do so in my teaching. If we look upon syphilis we will see that man's own act leads him to the place where he comes in contact with syphilis; it is the result of action.

Syphilis is that disease which corresponds to the effect of impure coition, of going where syphilis is, of coming in contact with those who have it. It is an action; it is not so with psora. Man does not seek it, he does not go where it is, he does not associate with those necessarily that have it. He may be exposed; but syphilis is the result of his own action, which is an impure fornication or adulteration which he knows better than to seek, and knows enough from his intelligence to avoid. Syphilis, then, is a result of action, although after once ultimated it may be perpetuated by accident. There is always a state and condition of man that precedes his action, and if syphilis corresponds to man's action; and there is a state prior to it, a diseased condition that precedes, that state must correspond to that which precedes action, which is thinking and willing.

Thinking and willing establishes a state in man that identifies the condition he is in. As long as man continued to think that which was true and held that which was good to the neighbour, that which was uprightness and justice, so long man remained upon the earth free from the susceptibility to disease, because that was the state in which he was created. So long as he remained in that state and preserved his integrity he was not susceptible to disease and he gave forth no aura that could cause contagion; but when man began to will the things that were the outcome of his false thinking then he entered a state which was the perfect correspondence of his interior. As are the will and understanding, so will be the external of man. As the life of man or as the will of man, so is the body of man, and as the two make one in this world, there is evolved from him an aura which is vicious in proportion to his departure from virtue and justice into evils. And long before the time of Noah's flood, which was an inundation that destroyed the evil ones that were upon the earth at that time, there was a manifestation, called leprosy, which was but the result of the dreadful profanity that took place in this period. A great many people suffered then from the violent aura of leprosy, whereas the natural disorder of the human race today is a milder form of psora upon a different race of people. If we had the same race upon the earth today we would have leprosy among them, as we now have the milder form of psora. The ancients referred to leprosy as an internal itch.

Hence this state, the state of the human mind and the state of the human body, is a state of susceptibility to disease from willing evils, from thinking that which is false and making life one continuous heredity of false things, and so this form of disease, psora, is but an outward manifestation of that which is prior in man. It was not due to actions of the body, as we find syphilis and sycosis to be, but due to an influx from a state, which progressed and established itself upon the earth, until we can see it as but the outward manifestations of man's very nature.

The human race today walking the face of the earth is but little better than a moral leper. Such is the state of the human mind at the present day. To put it another way, everyone is psoric. We know what leprosy means, and to say that the whole world is in a state of psora is no broader or narrower than to say that leprosy prevails today upon the face of the earth, but it prevails in a milder form, in the form of psora. A new contagion comes with every child. As psora piles up generation after generation, century after century the susceptibility to it increases. This is true of every miasm and true of all drugs. We find in the drugged world that those who have been mercurized become more susceptible to Mercury and are more easily poisoned by it. Those poisoned with Rhus are so sensitive to it that they cannot go within a whiff of it; those that have been poisoned in their earliest beginning with psora become more sensitive to it, so that in childhood the slightest whiff of it from their school friends will bring on a crop of vesicles between the fingers attended with the acarus.

Of course, some persons will say that the acarus is prior to the eruption, but they don't know that a healthy person will not be affected by the acarus. The miasm is simply evolved out of a state and the acarus is in turn its ultimate. It is the state that is prior, the itching is not prior. The human race becomes increasingly sensitive generation after generation to this internal state, and this internal state is the underlying cause which predisposes man to syphilis. If he had not psora he could not take syphilis; there would be no ground in his economy upon which it would thrive and develop.

The will and the understanding are prior to man's action. This is fundamental. The man does not do until he wills; he wills what he carries out. If man did what he did not will, he would be only an automation. He wills to go to a house of prostitution, or seeks for a prostitute with whom to copulate, and from her he takes the syphilitic miasm. This action of his will and this disease corresponds to the man. There is a state in which he thinks it only, in which he wills, but in which he has not yet arrived at the state in which he can act. First there was the thinking of falses and willing of evils, thinking such falses has led to depraved living and long for what was not one's own, until finally action prevailed. The miasms which succeeded psora were but the outward representations of actions, which have grown out of thinking and willing.

Psora is the oldest outward expression of the diseases of the human race representing this vital beginning and next exists that state that corresponds to action. Thinking, willing, and acting are the three things that make up the science of the life of the human race. Man thinks, he wills and he acts. Now, that aura which is given out from the human race at any period of its history is that which corresponds to the state of the human race. The children inherit it from their parents and carry it on and continue it. As the internal is so is the external, and the external cannot be except as the result of the internal.

The internal state of man is prior to that which surrounds him therefore, environment is not cause; it is only, as it were, a sounding board; it only reacts upon and reflects the internal. One who has the prior which is internal, may have that which can follow upon the external; it flows as it were from the internal and effect its forms upon the skin, upon the organs, upon the body of man Such is the influx and the inflowing is always in the direction of the least or no resistance; so that it is in the direction of man's affections, man's loves. Things flow in the direction he wants them to flow. Diseases correspond to man's affections, and the diseases that are upon the human race today are but the outward expression of man's interiors, and it is true if the diseases are such they represent the internal forces of man. Man hates his neighbour, he is willing to violate every commandment; such is the state of man today. This state is represented in man's diseases. All disease upon the earth, acute and chronic, are representations of man's internals. Otherwise he could not be susceptible, or could not develop that which is within him. The image of his own interior self comes out in disease.

This state has continued to progress, and it has accumulated and become complex. The original simple psora has added to it syphilis and sycosis, and these progress and have now effected a state, they have continued to effect a state in mankind, whereby the race is so susceptible to acute affections that many of our citizens have every little thing that comes along, and every little epidemic of influenza brings them down with an acute attack. This could not be but for the complications that a man has caused himself to get into, or has taken upon himself. This was not done in one generation, but has been accumulating upon the face of the earth so long as we have a history of man. Otherwise man would not be sick, for he should be a perfect animal in his animal nature.

Look at the perfection of all things put upon the earth; see the plants, how perfect they are; but man by his thinking evils and willing falses has entered upon a state wherein he has lost his freedom, his internal order, and is undergoing changes which the animal kingdom in its period, and the vegetable kingdom in its period, did not take on.

The miasms that are at the present day upon the human race are complicated a thousand fold by allopathic treatment. Every external manifestation of the miasm has in itself a tendency to straighten mankind, but the human race is being violently damaged and diseases are being complicated for the reason that these outward expressions are forced to disappear by the application of some violent or stimulating drug. At the present day, nobody will acknowledge that he had the itch in his childhood, until it is seen by some intelligent mother that it is wise to tell the doctor everything. The itch is looked upon as a disgraceful affair; so is everything that has a similar correspondence; because the itch in itself has a correspondence with adultery, only one is adultery as to internal and the other to externals, one succeeds the other. So it is with all miasms.

And now we have the great miasms before us to treat, as physicians, in all their complications. For instance, if a true sycotic gonorrhoea appears to us second hand it appears in its suppressed form, which is a thousand times worse than the original form. All the outward manifestations have been made to disappear. So it is with the external forms of psora, the vesicular and squamous eruptions, and all the outgrowths and outcroppings of psora. Every conceivable thing has been resorted to, to destroy its manifestations and the disease has grown and grown until nobody can tell what its outcome will be. How long can this thing go on before the human race will be swept from the earth with the results of the suppression of psora? From the suppression of psora we have cancerous affections, organic diseases of the heart and lungs, phthisis, and general destruction of the body. How long can it go on? If homoeopathy does not spread, if it does not establish its doctrines upon the earth so that sick folks can be headed under its principles, this threatening state and condition will increase. Allopathic physicians are multiplying rapidly, and they are all doing the same thing, even more so now than at the time of Hahnemann. It does seem as if homoeopathy had become a necessity, but the kind of homoeopathy that is preached in the majority of our schools will not check the progress of psora. The majority of the college teachers sneer at the doctrine of psora; they sneer at the miasms and continue in their efforts to establish homoeopathy upon an allopathic basis. Homoeopathy as taught in the colleges at the present day is simply an attempt to establish homoeopathy upon an allopathic basis, using allopathic names, calling chronic affections by different names, and treating diseases of organs by name. No study is made of psora, but allopathic books are their textbooks. Syphilis is not treated from cause to effect, but simply in the way of driving it back or holding it in abeyance, without any effort to permanently cure it. The patient is filled with Mercury, the Iodides and other strong drugs, drugs that are well known to subdue it temporarily by an allopathic effect.

Psora has progressed until it has become the most contagious of diseases, because the more complicated it becomes the more susceptible are our children to its beginnings, and its contagion adds to the old disease; and while it goes on the children become increasingly sensitive to the other miasms. The human race at the present day is intensely susceptible to psora, to syphilis and sycosis. "Psora," says Hahnemann, "became, therefore, the common mother of man's chronic diseases. It can be said that at least seven-eighths of the chronic maladies existing at the present day are due to psora."

True, if psora could be brought back in a series to its simple state the external of the body would become wonderfully bad to look upon, but the internal would be in a much better state. The vesicular eruptions that come are sometimes dreadful to look upon, horrible in proportion to the vanity of the patient, but these must be allowed to evolve themselves and then wonderful good comes to the economy. Hereditary states roll out in these manifestations, internal evils flow into external manifestations and homoeopathy continues to drive them outward and outward, thereby leaving the economy in a state of comparative freedom. Very commonly itch will not yield to the homoeopathic treatment immediately, because the action of the remedy is routing the heredity within, causing it to flow out more exteriorily into manifestations without. One who does not know this, of course, loses heart when his remedies do not at once wipe out the eruption. A sickly child may come out with eruptions, and if the child is treated properly the sickness will out into the eruption and that child will be cured from within out; and finally after much tribulation the outward trouble will pass away, carrying with it the internal trouble. So that when it is said that the appropriate remedy did not immediately wipe off the skin and make it smooth, and, therefore Zinc ointment or Sulphur ointment was resorted to, we see that it is a violation of law, and a wonderful damage to the patient.

Then Hahnemann gives a long list of cases with authorities, quotations and references which you should certainly look over. He also gives the symptoms that he collected while observing and investigating. It was the wonderful similarity between those symptoms when grouped together, representing an image of psora, and those symptoms representing, an image of Sulphur, which led Hahnemann to the use of Sulphur in psoric conditons. In psora we have the images of many remedies; all of the deep acting remedies have more or less something of the nature of psora.

Classroom Notes (Continued)

The three chronic miasmas, Psora, Sycosis and Syphilis are disease states, that are transferable. In each instance, there is something prior to the manifestations that we call the disease.

When we speak of the signs and symptoms of syphilis, we must remember that there is a state prior to syphilis or syphilis will not exist. It cannot come upon an individual unless conditions are suitable for it's development. In like way, Psora cannot exist except for a condition in mankind suitable for it's development.

Inheritance of Syphilis with Psora

1. Psora was the first and the other two miasmas came later. It is essential for us to inquire into that state of the human race that has been suitable for the development of Psora. There must have been a state of the human race suitable to the development of Psora. It cannot have come upon a perfectly healthy race. It will not exist in a perfectly healthy race. There must have been some sickness prior to this state.

2. If we look upon syphilis we will see that man's own act leads him to the place where he comes in contact with syphilis; it is the result of action. He may be exposed and infected by the *Tryponema pallidum*, but syphilis is the result of his own action, which is impure coitus or adulteration, which he knows better than to seek, and knows enough from his intelligence to avoid. There is always a state and condition of mind that precedes action, which is thinking and willing. Thinking and willing establishes a state in an individual that identifies the miasmatic state prior to the expression of miasmatic disease of that individual.

3. The will and the understanding are prior to man's action. This is fundamental. The man does not act until he wills. The miasma that succeeded Psora were but the outward representations of actions, which have grown out of thinking and willing.

4. When man began to will the things that were the out come of his false thinking. Thinking of such falses led to depraved living and longing for things not one's own, until action prevailed and then he entered a state that was the perfect correspondence of his interior. As are the will and understanding, so will be the external of man. Hence this state, the state of the human mind and the state of human

body, is a state of susceptibility to disease from willing evils, from thinking which is false and making life one continuous search of false things, and eventually this results in disease.

5.   Syphilis and sycosis are diseases that are due to the effect of impure coitus, after coming in contact with those who have it. If one wills to go to a house of prostitute or seeks multiple sex partners, it is because of faulty action of faulty will and understanding but this is not so with Psora. Man does not seek it, he does not go where it is, and he does not associate with those necessarily who have it.

6.   Psora is but an outward manifestation of that which is defective in human race. It is not due to the actions of the body, as we find Syphilis and sycosis to be, but due to an influx from a state, which has progressed and established itself upon the human race from generation to generation, until we can see it as the outward manifestations of man's very nature.

7.   To put it another way, everyone is Psoric. The human race becomes increasingly sensitive, generation after generation to this internal state, and this internal state is the underlying cause that predisposes man to Syphilis. If he did not have Psora, he could take Syphilis; there would be no ground in his internal state, upon which it would thrive and develop. The miasma has simply evolved out of a state and the disease is in turn its ultimate. It is the state that is prior to the disease. The itch bug is not prior.

8.   As long as the man continues to think, which was true and held which was good to the neighbor, which was upright and just, so long he remained upon the earth free from the susceptibility to disease. That was the state in which he was created. So long as he remained in that state and preserved his integrity he was not susceptible to disease. Thinking and willing establishes a state in man that identifies the condition in which he is.

9.   Thinking, willing and acting are the three things that make

up the science of the life of human race. Man thinks, he wills and he acts. Now, the aura which is given out from the human race at any period of its history, is which corresponds to the state of human race.

10. Diseases corresponds to man's affections, and the diseases that are upon the human race today are but, the outward expression of man's interior, and it is true if the disease are such that, they represent the internal forces of man. All diseases upon the earth, acute and chronic, are representations of man's interior. Otherwise he will not be susceptible. The image of his own interior self comes out in disease.

11. The original simple Psora has added itself to Syphilis and Sycosis, and have now effected a state, they have continued to effect state of mankind, whereby the race is so susceptible to acute affections that, many of our citizens have every little thing that comes along, and every little epidemic of influenza brings them down with an acute attack. Mankind by its thinking of evils and willing of falsies has entered upon a state where in it has lost its freedom.

12. How long can this thing go on before the human race will be swept from the earth with the results of the suppression of Psora? From the suppression of Psora we have cancerous affections, organic diseases of the heart and lungs, phthisis, and general destruction of the body. How long can it go on? The majority of the college teachers sneer at the doctrine of Psora; they sneer at the miasmas and continue in their efforts to establish Homeopathy upon an Allopathic basis. Homeopathy as taught in the colleges at the present day is simply an attempt to establish Homeopathy upon an Allopathic basis, using Allopathic names, calling chronic affections by different names, and treating diseases of organs by names. No study of Psora is made.

13. "Psora", says Hahnemann, "became, therefore, the common mother of man's chronic diseases. It can be said that at least seven eighth of the chronic maladies existing at the present day are due to Psora."

Hereditary states roll out in these manifestations, internal evils flow into external manifestations and Homeopathy continues to drive them outward and outward, thereby leaving the economy in a state of comparative freedom. Very commonly itch will yield to the Homeopathic treatment immediately, because the action of the remedy is routing the heredity within, causing it to flow out more exteriorly onto the skin. One who does not know this, of course, loses heart when his remedies do not at once wipe out the eruption.

14.   A sick child may come with eruptions, and if the child is treated properly the sickness will flow out into the eruption and that child will be cured from within to without and finally after much tribulation the outward trouble will pass away, carrying with it the internal trouble. So that when it is said that the appropriate remedy did not immediately wipe off the skin and make it smooth and, therefore Zinc ointment was resorted to, we see that it is a violation of law, and a woeful damage to the patient.

15.   True, if Psora could be brought back in a series to its simple state in an individual, the external of his body would become woefully bad to look upon, but the internal would be in a much better state. The vesicular eruptions that come are sometimes dreadful to look upon, but these must be allowed to evolve themselves and then wonderful good comes to the internal state.

LECTURE XX

Chronic Diseases—Syphilis

THERE are some generals that relate to this disease under homeopathic treatment. It can be found from books what to expect in this disease; for instance, the, different syphilitic eruptions in all their varied manifestations as to time and color. In regard to the prodromal period, it is well to remember that it is usually from twelve to fifteen days, but it is sometimes as late as 50 or 60 days. Some acute miasm or a bad cold, or a drug disturbing the economy, may prevent the external manifestations and prolong the prodromal period, but it is usually from 12-15 days, if in no way disturbed or interrupted. Now the prodromal period increases with the contagion of the various stages. This is an observation that you will be able to verify in homoeopathic practice, but one that the books will not give. The books speak of the primary contagion as the only contagion in connection with the syphilitic miasm, but let me tell you something. Suppose we assume that the syphilitic miasm is a disease that would run for a definite time, and suppose that an individual has gone through with the primary manifestation and is told by his physician that he can safely marry; if he marry, his wife becomes an invalid; but she does not go through the primary manifestations, the initial lesion and the roseola, but she has the syphiloderma and the symptoms which belong to the later stage of the disease. This disease is transferred from husband to wife, and it is taken up in the stage in which it then exists and from thence goes on in a progressive way. The woman catches it from the man in the stage in which he has it at the time of their marriage; she takes that which he has; if he has it in the advanced stage she takes it in that stage; she takes from him the stage he has to offer.

This is equally true of psora and sycosis. Such things never occur in the acute miasm, but the three chronic miasms have contagion in the form in which they exist at the time. The state is transferred, so that one in the advanced stages of psora will transfer to his good wife the psora which he has, and she takes it up and progress with it and adds it to her own, and it progresses in accordance with her peculiarities.

But the law of protection by dissimilars often comes in here and saves the wife's system from receiving a new infection of either syphilis, psora or sycosis. The disorders already present in her economy may be so wholly dissimilar that they protect her from contagion. Thus it is that a woman may have coition with a man that has sycosis in the form of gleet, and yet not have it indicated upon her; thus she may have protection against form of chancre. She may remain in contact with him as wife, and even have a child by him, and that child be black with syphilis, while she has no symptoms of syphilis. The reason of this is that the child is from the seed of the father and the mother only furnishes the groundwork.

There are plenty of physiological facts that demonstrate these things. I have seen several cases where the child was born black with syphilis, and have looked for the mother to come down with syphilitic symptoms, but no trace of it could be observed. When infection takes place in the primary stage there is no way of disguising it, but if it occurs in the secondary or tertiary stage there is really no way of detecting it immediately, because it goes on insidiously. If the husband has the primary sore it will manifest itself in the wife, but if he gives the disease to his wife in the tertiary stage, with every manifestation suppressed or passed by, then you will not be able to know whether she has taken the disease or not. We have already seen in studying the *Organon* that when the diseases are dissimilar to each other one repels the other; so that if the woman has something in her economy in the form of a chronic disease, perhaps a phthisical condition, she will be protected. The organic results are such that the body is overwhelmed with the disease that it already has, and hence she is protected. Dissimilars repel each other, and similars attract and cure each other. Yet if the dissimilar psoric manifestation is of a milder type, and can be substituted by the contagion, then the syphilitic condition comes in. To know the action of diseases upon each other is essential, because we see the principle of cure in how one disease affects another.

We learn much concerning the syphilitic miasm under the action of homoeopathic remedies. At the end of the prodromal period we may expect the chancre; at the end of about six weeks, more or less, we may expect the external manifestations, the roseola and other eruptions; soon succeeding these, at the time of their disappearance, or in connection with them, we have the mucous patches in the throat, ulcers in the throat, and finally the falling of the hair. These rapidly succeed each other, often being associated. These are the commonest outward manifestations of the earlier period of secondary syphilis; it is important to remember this. In weakly subjects these come on very feeble; in robust, vigorous constitutions these manifestations come on vigorously. Now it matters not whether the feeble constitution fails to throw these out, or whether because of drugs the constitution has been made feeble and thereby the manifestations are withdrawn when they have been thrown out. The state is the same, whether they are suppressed or withheld because of feeble constitution, *i.e.,* the disease is operating upon the internal, having a tendency to affect the organs that are of the interior man, the brain, the liver, the kidneys, the spleen, the heart and lungs, the tissue and the bones. As syphilis commences to occupy the interior tissues of man the periosteum, the bone and the brain are tissues that are sought out as the principal sites. If you will contrast that with psora you will see that the latter more commonly attacks the blood vessels and the liver and causes deposits beneath the skin, forming suppuration and boils. The syphilitic boil is not a true boil, it is a multiple tubercular mass most vicious in character.

If we observe the syphilitic miasm in its backward progress we will trace it back in its stages, supposing they had been suppressed. In the earlier state the homoeopathic treatment strikes at the root of the evil, and will take hold of that which would become latent, and will so turn things into order that the chancre that is painful will become painless, will continue on as a mild and harmless sore. The bubo will be hastened to suppuration when it would not otherwise suppurate. The mucous patches will be checked, the sore throat will be greatly relieved, so that the patient is made more comfortable in all of his manifestations. In this earlier state we do not see the backward progress in the form of ulcers, etc., but we see that the tendency of the homoeopathic remedy is, as it were, to quiet manifestations or subdue them, until the remedy has taken a deep and permanent hold of the economy, then they gradually subside.

So much for the action of homoeopathic remedies upon earlier manifestations. But now if we proceed to examine the very latest manifestations we will see an opposite state. If you take hold of a case that is very late, say an old case that has been five or ten years going the rounds, getting all sorts of vicious treatment, and the patient has those awful biparietal head pains, he is becoming weaker in mind, he is getting the tertiary manifestations in general, tendency to gummatous formations and deep-seated ulcerations, and is threatening to break down in health. You will find constitutional remedies can only restore him and cure him by bringing out external manifestations upon his body somewhere. Not that the primary sore will come back right away; he may never have it at all; but he will begin to have ulcerated sore throat, which may progress and eat all the soft tissues in view, including the soft palate. If this ulceration appears the bones that have been so painful and threatened to become necrosed will cease to be affected; the periostitis will subside. Iritis is likely to be a trouble-

or long years afterwards with tertiary symptoms. The proper remedy will immediately relieve this last appearing symptom, but the patient will say: "Doctor, I wish you would look in my throat; I have not had this trouble for a long time:' You see upon examining his throat a mucous membrane that has been sacrificed by the application of Nitric acid and other caustics, indurated, hard, gristly-like tissues that are infiltrated with gummatous deposits. Now, he is in a pickle, for just as sure as he lives that man will have to undergo much trouble if you save him from insanity. If you save him at all, so that he is worth living, these suppressed manifestations must come back, and they will come back under appropriate treatment.

Classroom Notes

Chronic Disease-Syphilis

1. As regard to the prodromal period, it is to remember that it is usually from twelve to fifteen days. It is sometimes as late as 50 or 60 days.

2. At the end of the prodormal period we may expect the chancre. At the end of about six weeks, more or less, we may expect external manifestations, the roseola and other eruptions; soon succeeding these, at the time of their disappearance, or in connection with them, we have the mucous patches in the throat, ulcers in the throat, and finally the falling of the hair.

3. These are the commonest outward manifestations of the earlier period of secondary Syphilis.

4. It is important to remember that in a weak subjects these symtoms come on very feeble; in robust, vigorous constitutions these manifestations come on vigorously.

5. Now it matters not whether the feeble constitution fails to throw these out, or whether because of drugs the constitution has been made feeble and thereby the manifestations are withdrawn when they have been thrown out. The state

is the same, whether they are suppressed or withheld because of feeble constitution, i.e., the disease is operating upon the internal, having a tendency to affect the organs that are of the interior man, the brain, the liver, the kidneys, the spleen, the heart and lungs, the tissues and the bones.

6.   As Syphilis commences to occupy the interior tissues of man, the periosteum, the bone and the brain are tissues that are sought out as the principal sites. If you will contrast this to sycosis, you will see that the latter, more commonly attacks the blood vessels and the liver and causes deposits beneath the skin, forming suppuration and boils. The syphilitic boil is not a true boil; it is a multiple tubercle, most vicious in character.

7.   Suppose we assume that the syphilitic miasma is a disease that will run for a definite time, and suppose that an individual had gone through the primary manifestations and is told by his physician that he can safely marry. His wife becomes an invalid. She does not go through the primary manifestations, the initial lesion and the roseola, but she has the syphiloderma and the symptoms that belong to the later stage of disease. This disease is transferred from the husband to wife. It is taken up in the stage in which it then exists and from there on it progress further. The woman catches from the man in the stage, in which he has it at the time of their marriage. She takes that which he has. If he has it in the advanced stage she takes in that stage. She takes from him the stage he has to offer.

8.   The state is transferred, so that one in the advanced stages of Syphilis will transfer to his good wife the Syphilis that he has. She takes it up and progresses with it and adds it to her own. It progresses in accordance with her peculiarities. She may remain in contact with him as wife, and even have a child by him. That child is black with Syphilis, while he has no symptoms of Syphilis. The reason is that the child is from the seed of the father and the mother only furnishes the groundwork.

9.   If we observe the syphilitic miasma in reprospective

manner, we will trace it back in its stages, supposing they had been suppressed. In the earlier state the Homeopathic treatment strikes at the root of the evil, and will take hold of that which will become latent, and will turn things into order. The chancre, which is painful will become painless, will continue on as a mild and harmless sore. The bubo will be hastened to suppuration when it will not otherwise suppurate. The mucous patches will be checked, the sore throat will be greatly relieved, and thus the patient is made more comfortable in all of his manifestations.

10. If you take up a case, which is five or ten years old, getting all sorts of vicious treatment, and the patient has those awful bi-parietal head pains. He is becoming weaker in mind. Then constitutional remedies can only restore him and cure him by bringing out external manifestations upon his body somewhere. Not always would the primary sore come back right away. In fact he may never have it at all; but he will begin to have ulcerated sore throat, which may progress and eat all the soft tissues in view, including the soft palate. If this ulceration appears the bones that have been so painful and threatened to become necrosed will cease to be affected; the periostitis will subside. Iritis is likely to be a troublesome symptom and may come with the secondary symptoms, or long years afterwards with tertiary symptoms. The proper remedy will immediately relieve this last appearing symptom, but the patient will say: "Doctor, I wish you will look in my throat; I have not had this trouble for a long time." Upon examining you see, his throat and mucous membrane that has been scarred by the application of Nitric acid and other caustics, tissues that are infiltrated with gummatous deposits. Now, he is in a pickle, for just as sure as he lives that man will have to undergo much trouble, if you save him from insanity, if you save him at all. These suppressed manifestations must come back, and they will come back under appropriate treatment.

LECTURE XXI

Chronic Diseases—Sycosis

IT is not generally known that there are two kinds of gonorrhoea, one that is essentially chronic, having no disposition to recovery, but continuing on indefinitely and involving the whole constitution in varying forms of symptoms, and one that is acute, having a tendency to recover after a few weeks or months. They are both contagious. There are also simple inflammations of the urethra attended with discharges which are not contagious, and thus we have simple inflammations of the urethra and specific inflammations of the urethra, and of the specific we have the two kinds I have mentioned, the chronic and acute. The books will treat of them as one disease, treat them in a class, and in a treatise on gonorrhoea we will have a description only of that which relates to the beginning, viz.; the discharge. The majority of the cases of gonorrhoea are acute, i.e., there is a period of prodrome, a period of progress and a period of decline, being thus in accordance with the acute miasms. The acute may really and truly be called a gonorrhoea, because about all there is of it is this discharge. If the suppressive treatment be resorted to in the acute, the system is sufficiently vigorous in most cases to throw off the after effects. The suppression cannot bring on the constitutional symptoms called sycosis. It cannot be followed by fig warts, nor constitutional states, such as anaemia. But while constitutional symptoms cannot follow the suppression of the acute miasm, they will follow suppression of the chronic miasm, and become very serious. Most of the cases of true sycosis that are brought before the physician at the present time are those that have been suppressed, and they are a dozen times more grievous than when in the primary stage.

In both the acute and chronic, the prodromal period is about the same, from eight to twelve days, and there is no essential difference between the discharge of the acute and chronic. It is a mucopurulent discharge, and may have all the appearances that any acute discharge of the urethra might take on. Any simple remedy confirms to the nature of the discharge itself will soon turn the acute miasm into a state of health, but it requires antisycotic remedies (remedies that confirm to the nature of sycosis) to turn the constitutional sycotic gonorrhoea into health. In the very earliest stage of the discharge it is not necessary to make a distinction; but after the disease progresses for weeks, it becomes necessary to make a distinction, and to follow the remedy that conformed to the more acute symptoms with the remedy that would be suitable in a sycotic constitution fully developed. Remedies are picked out for sycosis in the same way that the remedies are picked out in any miasmatic disease, viz., by making an anamnesis.

An anamnesis of all the sycotic cases which we have had enables us to look at the constitutional state of sycosis just in the same way as Hahnemann, by all anamnesis of psora, ascertained its nature and worked out the remedies that are similar in nature and action to psora. All medicines that are capable of producing the image of sycosis may be called anti-sycotics, but we can put it in this way also and say all those remedies are anti-sycotic which when given to a sycotic case in its advanced state are able to turn the disease backward, to reproduce the earlier forms and bring back the discharge. That is the practical way of demonstrating that a medicine is an anti-sycotic. When it conforms to the image of the miasm, it will turn the disease on its backward course. Those remedies that conform only to a particular part of the case are not deep enough nor similar enough to establish a return to earlier symptoms, and hence they are not truly anti-sycotic.

It is hardly necessary to go over a description of the acute form of gonorrhoea, but let us turn our attention solely to sycosis, recognizing it as a chronic miasm, or a disease whose first stage is a discharge from the urethra. These cases I have said are rare in proportion to the large number of cases of acute gonorrhoea, but the disease seems to be on the increase. Every busy physician will see a good many cases in women and children. Cases of gonorrhoea that have been suppressed by injections in the hands of the old school are considered ended, and soon after the discharge has stopped the sycotic patient may be told by his physician that he is a fit subject to marry as he has been cured. But it is not true, and he should delay marriage. It is not right for him to marry until the discharge has been brought back again, and he has been cured, by injections, because they only suppress, but by the indicated anti-sycotic. Only then may he marry a healthy wife, and she will continue healthy and bring forth healthy children.

You will never know until you get in practice how common it is for a wife to break down, in a year or eighteen months after marriage, with uterine trouble, with ovarian disease, with abdominal troubles, with all sorts of complaints peculiar to the woman; and you will then be surprised on going into the history of her husband (if you are permitted to do so) to discover that in his earlier life he had two or three attacks of gonorrhoea that were treated with Nitrate of Silver or by one of these prescriptions that are carried around in the vest pockets of vicious young men, by injections that are known to stop these discharges. You will not then be surprised if you learn that the man himself has never had a really genuine state of health since that gonorrhoeal discharge disappeared. You will look upon what followed that suppression in the man. You will observe what followed the contagion in the woman and to observe these closely constitutes an interesting study.

Sometimes it is so very severe in form, and the trouble comes so soon after the suppression, that there can be no doubt even in the mind of the man himself, that the trouble he is now suffering from relates to the suppression of that discharge. Sometimes they are latent and develop very gradually, and the blood becomes affected, the gradually increasing anaemia comes, the patient being pallid and waxy. What was said in relation to syphilis about contagion in the stage in which the individual has the disease is true in this disease, as also in psora. Here is a common instance. A sycotic patient has been "cured" as far as the discharge is concerned, and now marries for he is told that no harm can come hereafter but shortly afterwards his wife comes down with illness, whereas she had always been a healthy woman before. In the old school there is no recognition of a gonorrhoeal condition; nor could the homoeopathic physician be sure of this, except for his careful prescribing.

You take a man who has gone from ten to fifteen years with this sycotic trouble. He is waxy, subject to various kinds of fig warts, his lips are pale and his ears almost transparent; he is going into a decline; he has various kinds of manifestations, and these manifestations appear in numerous particulars that we call symptoms. The physician sits down and makes a careful study of the case, and if his perception of it is similar to some long acting, deep acting medicine, and he administers this medicine to the patient, the patient begins to improve. The treatment is kept up, and in the course of weeks or months the patient comes into the office and says: "Doctor, if I had exposed myself I should think I had an attack of gonorrhoea." Now, knowing the diseases get well in the reverse order of coining, you certainly cannot be surprised to hear this story.

On the other hand, however, the trouble may have manifested itself in other mucous membranes of the body, and thus saved the man from his waxiness; he is not so pallid when the condition becomes busy in another region. These catarrhal manifestations may be catarrhal conditions of the eyes, but are commonly catarrhs of the nose. It is not an uncommon thing for a nasal catarrh to be sycotic and to have existed only since the gonorrhoea was suppressed. The catarrh is located in the nose and posterior nares with thick, copious discharge, and in spite of local treatment it has been impossible to suppress it. When the constitution is vigorous enough it will keep up the discharge in spite of the different specific remedies that have been administered, but in constitutions that are feeble diseases are easily driven to the centre, leaving the outermost parts of man. So it is often the case that a man with a thick, yellowish-green discharge from the nose, after a dose of Calcarea, which is an anti-sycotic, one of the deepest in character, has his old discharge brought back, and he says: "Doctor, I am not able to account for this, for I have been nowhere but with my wife." It is time to sit down and tell that man that in his earlier life he had a gonorrhoea, and that its nature was sycotic; for if it had not been of a specific character, it could not have transferred itself to the man's economy, affecting in that way his nose; that it has disappeared from its new site under the action of a truly homoeopathic prescription, and the original discharge has been brought back, the trouble that he had in the first place. This must be explained to him, and you can now tell him that he is in a position to regain his health, to become well, to get rid of his catarrh; but that if he meddles with that discharge from the penis he will never recover. Just this kind of a case has been seen so often that there it is no longer a doubt about it.

It is in the nature of gonorrhoea to go to the surface in the earlier stage, and so when the catarrh comes on in vigorous constitutions soon after the suppression of the discharge from the urethra it may locate itself in the nose, but if the catarrh does not come on soon the constitution is too weak for the catarrh to represent the disease, and it will be represented on deeper tissues. Bright's disease may come, breaking down of the lungs, breaking down of the liver, rheumatic affection of the worst form, finally killing the patient. It is only in the earlier stages that it becomes catarrhal. The man thinks he is cured and he has escaped the outward manifestations because his constitution is not very vigorous, but the disease goes on into an advanced state until it attacks the blood and he becomes anaemic.

Now, if in this condition he marry, his wife does not get the catarrhal state, because the contagion is contracted in the bladder trouble, but she gets the anaemic state. You may call it a secondary state if you like, but it is really the more interior form of the disease. From this anaemic state it spreads into all functions of the body. The woman does not get the catarrhal state, because the contagion is contracted in the woman at the stage which the husband has reached. If he has passed the catarrhal stage, what she gets is beyond the catarrhal state. She gets fibrinous condition, inflammation of the uterus and the soft tissues, or low grade changes in the kidneys. She may go on and have any of the peculiar constitutional diseases that the woman of today is subject to. It is rather strange that it affects the soft tissues and not the bones. Syphilis affects the soft tissues and the bones. Psora affects the whole economy, nothing escapes; it causes a general breakdown.

Sometimes in the man it does not take the catarrhal form, but produces inflammation of the testes, or it may affect the rectum. Again, if you go to the bedside of a man who has used strong injections for the purpose of suppressing a gonorrhoeal discharge, and you find him in bed writhing and turning, tossing and twisting with the pains, and the only relief for him is to keep in continual motion; the pains are tremendous, they are rending and tearing from head to foot; if he can get up he will walk the floor night and day. There is seldom much swelling with this rheumatism; it seems to be along the sheath of the nerves and is relieved by motion. The superficial physician will say, here is a patient relieved by motion, here is a case for Rhus. You give Rhus, and then find it does not do a single thing for the man; but remember, when you have studied sycosis in its innermost nature, Rhus is not an anti-sycotic remedy and will not help this patient in his restlessness; it will not help his awful distress and anxiety. This state will go on, and when it has attacked him so violently his tendons will begin to contract, they will shorten, the muscles of the calves will become sore, the muscles of the thighs will become so sore that they cannot be touched or handled; sometimes there is infiltration of the muscles and hardness, and this soreness extends to the bottom of the feet so that it is impossible for the patient to walk. He is compelled to sit or lie or crawl around on his hands and knees, so violent are some cases. These cases will go on for years. I have known external applications of the allopathic physician to be applied to these sore feet and limbs for weeks and months and even years, and yet they give no relief; but a correct prescription made by a homoeopath, carefully taking in account and covering the whole nature of sycosis, will take the soreness out of the feet and bring back the gonorrhoeal , discharge. The return of the old symptoms means recovery. When the discharge comes back the relief of these horrible symptoms comes, and do not consider any patient cured until the discharge is brought back.

With reference to the woman, in whom you know that the contagion has taken place in the stage in which it existed in the husband, supposing she has inflammation of a fibrinous character and goes into the very worst forms of anaemia, with all the sallowness and waxiness and patchy condition of the skin and the withering and the organic troubles, if a homoeopathic prescription be made that is truly anti-sycotic you need not expect that a gonorrhoeal discharge will appear in her case; it is not necessary, she can get well without it. If she had no discharge she can get well without its return. The reverse order of the symptoms in her case means only the reverse order of those she has had. She may not have had the primary, but all that that patient has had she must go back through, stage by stage and symptom by symptom. The woman is the most grievous sufferer; she is an innocent person, and when there are anaemic conditions and a going down steadily in the wife that has come on a few years after marriage you should always be suspicious of this disease, at least do not allow it to pass unless you have made a suitable investigation of the matter. Send for the husband, talk to him quietly, tell him you want to know whether he has gone through any of the specific diseases in his younger days that it shall be considered in confidence. When you are the family physician that must be done.

With fear and trembling he will likely tell you the whole story; he has gone into his marriage with a degree of innocence, because he was advised by his physician that what he has had will not affect his wife. When you have discovered this state in the family, watch their children; they will be few for sycosis very commonly makes a woman sterile, or if she has a few children you will find in them a strong tendency to marasmus in the first year, or in the first or second summer a strong tendency to consumption, or you will find a withering, old appearance of the face. Anyone of these three miasms may predispose this child to these things, but when the child is waxy and anaemic, is accustomed to have lienteric stools, has no digestion, when every hot spell brings on complaints that look like cholera-infantum, and it does not grow, does not thrive, you have a right to suspect it is a sycotic case, for sycosis is the most frequent cause.

This disease, you see, does not manifest itself by many eruptions, except those of a warty character; it does not manifest itself by eruptions like syphilis and psora, but operates by bringing about a rheumatic state and an anaemic condition of the blood. It takes hold of the blood first and conforms to the subjects who are advanced in deep-seated troubles, subject to epithelioma. They are especially subject to Bright's disease and to acute phthisis. If they have pneumonia, it is likely to end in a breakdown of some sort in the lungs. If they have any acute disease of a prolonged character, like typhoid, the recovery is always slow.

Manifestly it is a good thing to know the history of a patient, all the peculiarities of the life of a patient. It is important to know whether that patient is syphilitic or sycotic. You know that everybody is psoric, but those that have lived a proper life have escaped the two contagious diseases which man acquires in the first place by his own seeking. When a patient has gone to the end of typhoid or some lingering disease, you know that he is psoric, but if you also know that he is syphilitic, or that he is sycotic, you can conduct his convalescence into a speedy recovery, and if he denies these things you may be puzzled. The sycotic patient may go into a state of do-nothing and decline at the end of a typhoid fever; convalescence will not be established, he will lie with an aversion to food; he does not react, he does not repair, there is no tissue-making, no assimilation; there is no vitality, he lies in a sort of semi-quiescent state; there is no convalescing in the matter. If you know he is a sycotic patient, he must have an anti-sycotic remedy, and then he will begin to rally. If a syphilitic patient, he must have an anti-syphilitic remedy. If neither of these miasms are present, a remedy looking towards his psoric state will cause him to rally. The nature of these cases must be kept in view, you must remember that these chronic miasms are present in the economy and after an acute illness very often have to be fought. If this is not known, many patients will gradually sink and die for apparent want of vitality to convalesce.

Of course, the anti-sycotic treatment for the infant will bring back, as you will readily see, only that stage which the infant began with. It will not bring out a discharge in the infant. The infant has only the interior nature of the disease, and has not the primary and outermost forms of it. You will also remember another thing, that these infants when they grow up are increasingly sensitive to sycosis; that they are already prepared for a sycotic gonorrhoea whenever the first exposure comes. The susceptibility is laid by his inheritance, just as the susceptibility to psora is laid by our parents and the susceptibility to syphilis is laid by our parents. Man can only have one attack in his natural lifetime of one of the three chronic miasms; a man cannot take syphilis twice, he cannot take sycosis twice, he cannot take psora twice. This is not known; a man when asked how many times he has had gonorrhoea will say: "About half a dozen times;" but only one of these was sycotic. The sycotic constitution cannot be taken a second time. One attack gives immunity to that person forever after. The offspring becomes increasingly susceptible to all the miasms the more they become developed in the human race. The more they become complicated with each other the more the human race becomes susceptible to acute and epidemic diseases. Now, you have a general survey of the chronic miasms.

Classroom Notes

Chronic Disease—Sycosis

1. The *acute* Sycosis may really and truly be called Gonorrohea, because all that is there to it is discharge.
2. In both the acute and chronic, the prodromal period is approximately the same, from eight to twelve days.
3. There is no essential difference between the discharge of the acute and chronic. It is a *muco-purulent discharge*, and may have all the appearances that any acute discharge of the urethra might take on.
4. Any simple remedy that confirms to the nature of the discharge itself will soon turn the acute miasm into a state of health.
5. It requires *anti-sycotic remedies* (remedies that confirm to the nature of sycosis) to turn the constitutional sycotic gonorrhoea into health.
6. All medicines that are capable of producing the image of Sycosis may be called anti-sycotics. We can put it in this way also and say all those remedies are anti-sycotic, which when given to a sycotic case in its advanced state are able to turn disease backward, to reproduce the earlier forms and bring back the discharge. That is the practical way of demonstrating that a medicine is anti-sycotic.
7. Cases of gonorrhoea that have been suppressed by injections, in the hands of the old school are considered cured. After the discharge has stopped the sycotic patient is told that he is a fit subject to marry as he has been cured. But it is not true, and he should delay marriage. It is not right for him to marry until the discharge has been brought back again, and he has been cured, not by injections, because they only suppress, but by the indicated anti-sycotic. Only then he may marry a healthy wife, and she will continue healthy and bring forth healthy children.

8.   You will never know until you get in practice, how common
      it is for a wife to break down, in a year or eighteen months
      after marriage, with *uterine trouble*, with ovarian disease,
      with *abdominal troubles*, with all sorts of *complaints pecu-*
      liar to the *woman*. You will then be surprised going on, into
      the history of her husband. You will look upon what fol-
      lowed that suppression in he man. You will observe what
      followed the contagion in the woman and to observe these
      constitutes an interesting study.

9.   Sometimes these are latent and develop very gradually. The
      blood becomes affected, then gradually increasing *anemia*
      comes, the patient becomes *pallid and waxy*. What was said
      in relation to Syphilis about contagion in the stage, in which
      the individual has the disease is true in this disease, as also
      in Psora.

10.   The treatment is kept up, and in course of weeks or months
      the patient comes into the office and says: "*Doctor, if I had*
      exposed myself I think I had an attack of gonorrhoea". Now
      knowing the disease gets well in the reverse order of com-
      ing, you certainly cannot be surprised to hear this story.

11.   These *catarrhal manifestations* may be catarrhal conditions
      of the *eyes*, but are commonly catarrhs of the *nose*. It is not
      an uncommon thing for a nasal catarrh to be sycotic and to
      have existed only since, the gonorrhoea has been sup-
      pressed.

12.   When the constitution is vigorous enough it will keep up
      the discharge in spite of the different specific remedies that
      have been administered. In constitutions that are feeble, dis-
      eases are easily driven to center, leaving the outermost parts
      of man.

13.   It is in the nature of Gonorrhoea to go to the surfae in the
      earlier stage, and so when the catarrh comes on in vigorous
      constitutions soon after the suppression of the discharge
      from the urethra it may locate itself in the nose. If the
      catarrh does not come on soon the constitution is too weak

for the catarrh to represent the disease, and it will be represented on deeper tissues. *Bright's disease* may come, breaking down the *lungs*, breaking down the *liver*, *rheumatic affection* of the worst form and finally killing the patient. It is only in the earlier stages that it becomes catarrhal. Man thinks he is cured and he has escaped the outward manifestations untill it attacks the blood and he becomes anaemic.

14.   So it is often the case that a man with a thick, yellowish-green discharge from the nose, after a dose of Calcarea, which is an anti-sycotic, one of the deepest in character, has his old gleety discharge brought back, and he says: "*Doctor, I am not able to account for this, I have been nowhere but with my wife.*" It is time to sit down and tell that man that in his earlier life he had a gonorrhoea, and that its nature was sycotic; for it had not been of a specific character, it could not have transferred itself to the man's economy, affecting in that way his nose. That it has disappeared from its new site under the action of a truly Homeopathic prescription, and the original discharge has been brought back. This must be explained to him, and you can now tell him that he is in a position to regain his health, to become well, to get rid of catarrh; but that if he meddles with that discharge from the penis he will never recover.

15.   The women do not get the catarrhal state, because the contagion is not contracted in the woman at the stage, which the husband has reached. If husband has passed the catarrhal stage, what she gets is beyond the catarrhal state. She gets *fibrinous condition, inflammation of the uterus* and the soft tissues, or low grade *changes in the kidneys*. She may go on and have any of the peculiar constitutional diseases that the woman of today is subject to. It is rather strange that it affects the soft tissues and not the bones. Psora affects the whole internal state, nothing escapes; it causes a general breakdown.

16.   You go to the bedside of a man, who uses strong injections for the purpose of suppressing a gonorrheal discharge. You

find him in bed writhing and turning, tossing and twisting with the pains, and the *only relief* for him is to *keep in continual motion*; the pains are tremendous. They are rending and tearing from head to foot; if he can get up he will walk the floor night and day. There is seldom much swelling with this rheumatism. Pain seems to be along the sheath of the nerves and is relieved by motion. This state will go on, and since it has attacked him so violently his tendons will begin to contract. They will shorten. The muscles of the calves will become sore. The muscles of the thighs will become so sore that they cannot be touched or handled. Sometimes there is infiltration of the muscles and hardness, and this soreness extends to the bottom of the feet so that it is impossible for the patient to walk. Carefully taking in account and covering the whole nature of sycosis, if you prescribe an anti-sycotic then it will take the discharge. The return of the old symptoms means recovery. When the discharge comes back, the relief from these horrible symptoms comes, and do not consider any patient cured until the discharge is brought back.

17.   With reference to the woman, in whom you know that the contagion has taken place in the stage in which it existed in her husband, supposing she has inflammation of fibrinous character. If in such a case a Homeopathic prescription is made that is truly anti-sycotic you need not expect that a **gonorrhoeal** discharge will appear in her case; it is not necessary, she can get well without it.

18.   When you have this sycotic state in the family, watch their children. They will be few, for sycosis very commonly makes a *woman sterile*, or if she has a few children you will find in them a strong tendency to *marasmus* in the first year, or in the first or second summer a strong tendency *to consumption*, or you will find a withering, old appearance of the face. Any of these three miasmas may predispose the child to those things. But when the child is *waxy* and *anaemic*, is accustomed to have *lientric stools*, has improer

digestion, when every hot spell brings on complaints that look like *cholera-infantum*. It does not grow, does not thrive, you have a right to suspect it is a sycotic case, for Sycosis is the most frequent cause.

19. Syeotic disease, you see, does not manifest itself by many *eruptions, except those of warty character*. It does not manifest itself by eruptions like Syphilis and Psora, but operates by bringing about a *rheumatic state* and an *anaemic condition* of the blood. It takes hold of the blood. It takes hold of the blood first and conform to the subjects who are advanced in deep-seated troubles, subject to *epithelioma*. They are especially subject to *Bright's disease* and to *acute phthisis*. If they have *pneumonia*, it is likely to end in a breakdown of some sort in the lungs. If they have any acute disease of a prolonged character, like *typhoid*, the recovery is always slow.

Why must we know the Miasma?

1. Manifestly it is a good thing to know the history of a patient, all the peculiarities of the life of the patient. It is important to know whether that patient is Syphilitic or Sycotic.

2. You know that everybody is Psoric, but those who have lived a proper life have escaped the two contagious diseases, which man acquires in the first place by his own seeking.

3. If a patient has gone to the end of typhoid or some lingering disease, you know that he is Psoric. But if you also know that he is Syphilitic or Sycotic, you can conduct his convalescence into a speedy recovery.

4. If he denies these things you may be puzzled. The sycotic patient may go into a state of do-nothing and decline at the end of a typhoid fever. Convalescence will not be established. He will lie with to aversion to food. He does not react. He does not repair. There is no tissue regeneration, no assimilation. There is no vitality, he lays in a semi-quiescent state; there is no convalescing in the matter.

5. If you know he is a sycotic patient, he must have an anti-sycotic remedy, and then he will begin to rally.

6. If such a patient is syphilitic, he must have an anti-syphilitic remedy.

7. If neither of these miasma is present, a remedy looking towards his psoric state will cause him to rally.

8. The nature of these cases must be kept in view. Remember these chronic miasmas are present in the internal state and after an acute illness very often have to be fought. If this is not known, many patients will gradually sink and die for apparent want of vitality to convalescence.

9. Of course, the anti-sycotic treatment for the infant will bring back, as you will readily see, only that stage which the infant began with. It will not bring out a discharge in the infant. The infant has only the interior nature of the disease, and has not the primary and outermost forms of it.

10. Remember one thing, these infants when they grow up they are increasingly sensitive to Sycosis. They are already prepared for a sycotic gonorrhoea whenever the first exposure comes.

11. The susceptibility is laid by his inheritance, just as our parents lay the susceptibility to Psora and Syphilis.

12. The more the human race becomes susceptible to all the miasmas the more they become complicated with each other the more the human race becomes susceptible to acute and epidemic diseases.

    Now, you have a general survey of the chronic miasmas.

LECTURE XXII

Disease and Drug Study in General

PART of your study should be to bring before the mind, as fully as possible, the diseases that the human race is subject to. This cannot be done to any great extent from Old School books, as they do not treat of psora, syphilis and sycosis in such a way as to bring the image of the disease before the mind, and only in a limited way the acute miasms are so brought before the mind. The diagnostic or pathognomonic symptoms are brought out for the purpose of distinguishing one disease from the other, but not with the idea of bringing the image of the disease before the mind that it may look like some remedy recorded in the Materia Medica, because that is not the allopathic physicians way of prescribing. It is important to go over the great bulk of the psoric symptoms that Hahnemann has given to obtain as perfect an image as possible of the disease psora. If we take the *Chronic Diseases* and go over them, writing, out opposite every symptom that Hahnemann has mentioned as psoric all the remedies that have been found from provings to correspond to these disease symptoms, we shall have before the mind a list of the anti-psoric remedies. It is a good exercise and a good way of preparing for the study of Materia Medica.

Try to master this: Diseases must not be looked upon from a few symptoms that the patient may possess but from all the symtoms that the whole human race brings out. It is just as improper to look upon psora from a few symptoms as it is to look upon a remedy from a few symptoms. Just as you see the image of a remedy from all the symptoms, including the peculiar symptoms, so psora must be considered from its characteristics, the features that constitute psora. Remedies are adjusted as to appearance; the appearances of the remedy expressed in symptoms must be adjusted to the appearances of the disease expressed in symptoms. When you have finished psora, take up sycosis, and spend much time in gathering together all the symptoms that sycotic patients have felt, all their suffering and all the ultimates. Group them as one, and look upon them as one miasm. Then go to the Materia Medica again and make an anamnesis. Take each symptom and place opposite it all the remedies that have produced that symptom. You can readily see that the remedies that run through most strongly will be antisycotic remedies, *i.e.,* the remedies that have the essentials of the disease or the nature of sycosis in them.

In the same way make an anamnesis of syphilis. By these means you will bring before your mind the three chronic diseases of the human race, and when this is accomplished in a general way you will be prepared to enter upon their treatment. But remember that the symptoms, when it comes to prescribing for a chronic patient, constitute the whole basis of the prescription; we have not other. We may theorize as much as we have a mind to, but when it comes to the actual application the symptoms must guide to the remedy. There are, however, a good many different ways of looking at the symptoms. It is a very easy thing to become confused over the symptoms and fall into error by taking symptoms that are unimportant. Your study in the Materia Medica will illustrate how you must study disease, as the plan of studying the Materia Medica for the purpose of bringing the image of a remedy before the mind is the plan we must adopt in studying a disease. The physician who can only hold in his memory the symptoms of a disease or a remedy will never succeed as a homoeopath. He has not taught himself to think, he has only a mass of particulars, and nothing to tie to. There is no order. It is like a mob.

Here I want to read you a note of Hahnemann's. "Should it, however, be thought sometimes necessary to have names for diseases, in order to render ourselves intelligible in a few words to the ordinary classes when speaking of a patient, let none be made use of but such as are collective. We ought to say, for instance, that a patient has a species of chorea, a species of dropsy, a species of nervous fever, a species of ague," etc. It will lead the mind into heresay if one gets into the custom of speaking from appearances and naming diseases according to the old way. The homoeopathic physician must avoid thinking that way. One who has been in the habit of thinking that way must make a great effort to keep the mind from running in that groove. Of course, it would be folly to talk to an old school physician or to a patient in any other words and we can talk to them so, for the sake of conversing but we must know when we speak in such a way that it is only an appearance.

This now brings us to paragraph 83, which takes up the study and examination of the patient and the qualifications necessary for comprehending the image of a disease. You have probably by this time come to the conclusion that an old school prescriber, and perhaps the majority of such as call themselves homoeopaths at the present time, are perfectly incompetent to examine a patient, and therefore incompetent to examine homoeopathy, to test it, so as to say whether there is anything in it or not. They have every element of failure and no element of success. It is impossible to test homoeopathy without learning how to get the disease image so before the eye that the homoeopathic remedy can be selected. What a natural thing it would be for an allopathic physician to say: "I am going to test homoeopathy. This patient has a case of vomiting, and I will give Ipecacuanha because it produces vomiting." So he gives Ipecacuanha, and the patient keeps on vomiting. He has tested homoeopathy and it is no good! That is the way tests are usually made. I have had physicians tell me that they have tested homoeopathy and it failed; but I know that it was not homoeopathy that failed but the physician who failed. Whenever failure comes it is a failure of the physician and not of the law. This is about the kind of a test that is made today in this enlightened day and age of the world. They have neither the knowledge nor the state of mind to make a test. They do not know what to observe, or how to select a remedy. If we should look up all the remedies that have vomiting we would find a pretty good list, but to make use of that list the mind must be prepared to see which one in it is similar to this individual patient.

> "The examination of a particular case of disease, with the intent of presenting it in its formal state and individuality, only demands on the part of the physician an unprejudiced mind, sound understanding, attention and fidelity in observing and tracing the image of the disease, I will content myself in the present instance with merely explaining the general principles of the course that is to be pursued, leaving it to the physician to select those which are applicable to each particular case."

The first statement is that the physician must be of unprejudiced mind. Where are you going to find such a person? If that is essential there is almost nobody that can examine a case for the purpose of finding a remedy for that case. An unprejudiced mind! At the present day there is almost no such thing as an unprejudiced mind. Go out among the doctors who profess to practice homoeopathy and you will find they are full of prejudice. They will at once commence to tell you what they believe; one believes one thing and another thing; they all have varying kinds of belief. This does not come from a question of fact, but it comes from what each man has laid down as fact. What each man wants to be so, in his view, is so. That establishes in his mind a state of prejudice, and as no two agree there are many, different opinions, the majority of which must be false. Go into anything that you have a mind to and you will find man full of prejudice. This state of prejudice exists in the examination of a patient. The physician goes to the patient prejudiced as to his own theories. He has own ideas as to what constitutes the correct method of examination, and so he does not examine the patient for the purpose of bringing out the truth, the whole truth and nothing but the truth. His prejudices lead him to snap the patient up as soon as he begins to tell his story. He will thump him all over, from head to foot, and then tell him what is the matter with him. A prescription that has no earthly relation to the constitutional state of the patient follows, but no examination has really been made.

It might readily and truthfully be said that the true man has no prejudices. It is certain that the true man is one freest from prejudices, one who can listen, who can examine evidence and who can meditate. What would we think of a judge who would go into a case with strong prejudice? The law provides that a judge cannot sit in judgment over his brother or over his wife, or over his other relatives. In a homoeopathic physician an unprejudiced mind can only be attained by learning all the truth and all the doctrines of homoeopathy. If a physician goes in with prejudice for a certain potency or a certain disease, or a prejudice against certain principles, he is not in a rational state, he is not in freedom with the patient and he goes into the examination in ignorance, and if he cannot free himself from prejudice he cannot prescribe. If a man has arrived at a degree of sound understanding concerning the doctrines of homoeopathy, concerning the doctrines of potentization, concerning the doctrines that relate to chronic and acute diseases, concerning the Materia Medica, he goes into it with full freedom, with an intention to examine the case in all its length and breadth, and to listen patiently. He listens to the friends of the patient and he observes without prejudice, with wisdom and with judgment. He must go into the case without forming any judgment whatever until all the witnesses have told their tale and all the evidence is before him. Then he commences to study the whole case. That is doing it without prejudice and for this a sound understanding is necessary, with a clear knowledge of all things relating to the subject and to all of his duties.

If an allopathic physician was to come in and listen to the long examination of a case by a homoeopath he would want to know what it was all about. He does not see anything in it, because he has not a knowledge of true materia medica. The homoeopath's purpose is to transfer a man's sickness to paper and so find the, image of the sickness in the Materia Medica. The allopathic physician could not do that; he could not put the image of the sickness on canvas so that he could fit the picture to the Materia Medica, for he would not know one of our medicines with which to compare it. The unprejudiced mind then comes from sound understanding, and a sound understanding comes from education. The education we are now talking about is an education in homoeopathy, becoming acquainted with all the doctrines step by step. After being taught how to give attention and what to give attention to fidelity is necessary. This faithfulness would never be shown by one who had not removed all his prejudices by opening his mind to the principles and doctrines. Here we work together; we all work after the same fashion. Take everyone of the students that goes through here for a year, and you will find that he has the ways of the school and carries the stamp of the school. Just as the stamp of Harvard or the stamp of Yale is upon every student that comes from either of these institutions so the stamp of the Post Graduate School is upon every student that goes through its curriculum with faithfulness and earnestness.

What we are now about to consider is the plan for the faithful and careful examination of a case. It is our purpose to cure the case, and it is necessary for this purpose to bring the patient's symptoms in the very best possible way before the mind. This is a long and tedious study, and there are many difficulties in the way. Disease must be brought out in symptoms, with the end of its becoming a likeness of some remedy of the Materia Medica. All the diseases known to man have their likeness in the Materia Medica, and the physician must become so conversant with this art that he may perceive this likeness. You will find at first it is not an easy matter and that, to become expert, requires the continual application of patience. All the senses must be on the alert in

Classroom Notes

Disease and Drug Study in General

1. As a part of your study, it should be as much as possible, to bring before mind, the diseases that human race is subjected to. (The study of Miasm).

2. **Try to master this:** Disease must not be looked upon from a few symptoms that the patient may possess but from all the symptoms that the human race brings out.

3. **Remedies are adjusted as to appearance:** The appearance of the remedies expressed in symptoms must be matched with to the appearance of the disease expressed in symptoms.

4. We may theorize as much as we have in mind, but when it comes to actual application the symptoms must be the guide to a remedy.

The Plan of Studying: 'The Materia Medica' (For the purpose of bringing the image of a remedy before the mind)

(a) It is important to go over the great bulk of the Psoric symptoms that Hahnemann has given to obtain, as perfect an image as possible of the disease, Psora.

(b) Write out opposite every symptom that Hahnemann has mentioned as Psoric, all the remedies that have been found from provings correspond to these Psoric symptoms. We shall have before the mind, a list of the anti-Psoric remedies. That is to say, these remedies have the essential of the disease or the nature Psora in them.

(c) When you have finished Psora, take up Sycosis, and spend some time in gathering together all the symptoms that Sycotic patients have felt, all their sufferings and all their pathologies. Group them as one and look at them as one miasma.

(d)   Then take each symptom and place opposite it all the remedies that have produced those symptoms. You can readily see that the remedies that run through most strongly, will be anti-sycotic remedies, that is to say the remedies that have essentials of the disease or nature of Sycosis in them.

(e)   In the same way, study Syphilis.

[Para: 83]

Examine every case of a disease with the intention of knowing the *individuality*.

This requires the physician to have:

1.   An *unprejudiced* mind;
2.   *Sound understanding*; and
3.   Attention and faithfulness in *observing* and *tracing* the image of disease.

It is impossible to test Homeopathy without learning how to get the disease image before the eyes. Thus the Homeopathic remedy can be selected.

If a physician goes in with prejudice for certain potency or a certain disease or a prejudice against certain principles, he is not in freedom of mind and spirit. If a physician cannot free himself from prejudice (or try) he cannot prescribe well.

————————————

Lecture XXIII

The Examination of the Patient

§ 84. The patient details his sufferings; the persons who are about him relate what he has complained of, how he has behaved himself, and all that they have remarked in him. The physician sees, hears and observes with his other senses whatever there is changed or extraordinary in the patient. He writes all this down in the very words which the latter and the persons around him make use of. He permits them to continue speaking to the end without interruption, except where they wander into useless digressions, taking care to exhort them at the commencement to speak slowly that he may be enabled to follow them in taking down whatever he deems necessary.

ONE of the most important things in securing the image of a sickness is to preserve in simplicity what the patient tells us in his own way unless he digresses from the important things and talks about things that are foolish and not to the point; but as long as he confines his information to his own sufferings, let him tell it in his own way without interruption and in the record use his own language, only correcting his grammatical errors for the purpose of procuring the record as perfect as possible. If you use synonyms be sure that they are synonyms and cannot be perverted. Of course, when the woman speaks of her menstrual period as "monthlies" or as her "show," the more suitable medical term is "menses," which is a synonym for those expressions, and is more expressive than her own way of calling it "a show". So in general terms you can substitute terms of expression so long as you do not change the idea. Of course, the changing of "legs" into "limbs" if you feel like making such a change is not a change of thought, but be sure in making a change it is not a change of thought.

It is one of the most important things in forming the record of a patient to be able to read it at a subsequent examination, without being disturbed by the repeated statements of the patient. If you write a record in consecutive sentences, you will be so confused when hunting out the symptoms of the patient that you will be unable to form an image of that sickness in the mind. It is truly impossible when the mind is full with the effort at hunting cut something to listen with proper and concentrated attention. You should divide your page in such a manner that when the patient is talking to you about this thing and that thing and the other thing of her symptoms, you can with one glance of the eye look down over the page of the record and see everything there is in that page. If your record is not so arranged, it is defective. Now, a record can be so arranged by dividing the page into three columns, the first of which contains the dates and prescriptions, the second the emphatic symptoms or headings and the third things predicated of the symptoms, thus:

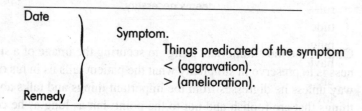

```
Date      ⎫
          ⎪   Symptom.
          ⎬   Things predicated of the symptom
          ⎪   < (aggravation).
          ⎪   > (amelioration).
Remedy    ⎭
```

After the patient has detailed his sufferings in his own way and you have gone through them and discovered all the things that you can predicate of his symptoms then you can proceed to make enquiry of some one who has been with this patient. In a study like this with most of our private patients there has been a nurse, sometimes only a sister or a mother or a wife, who has been observing all the sick individual has complained of. "The persons who are about him relate what he has complained of, how he has behaved himself, and all that they have remarked in him." Now, this should be listened to with great care. It is more important in this instance to decide whether the observer is over anxious, if a wife whether she is not frightened concerning her husband and so intermingles many of her notions and fears, which you must accept with discretion. Get the nurse, if possible, to repeat the exact words of the patient. If such a thing can be done in acute sufferings it is worth more than the words or expressions of the nurse, the wife for instance, because the more interested and anxious the person is the less likely she will be to present a truthful image, not that she wants to deceive, but she is dreadfully wrought up and the more she thinks of what he has said the greater his sufferings appear to her, and she exaggerates them. It is important to have the statement from one who is disinterested. Two or three of the observers who are intelligent having been consulted and their statements recorded, the physician then notes his own observations. He should describe the urine if there is anything peculiar about that, but if the urine and stool are normal he need not care about the description of these.

It has been the study for hundreds of years to find the best way to question witnesses in court, and as a result they have settled upon certain rules for obtaining evidence. Homoeopathy also has rules for examining the case that must be followed with exactitude through private practice. Among pupils who have been taught here, I know some who have merely memorized and some have not even memorized but have fallen away. These students are violating everything they have been taught; they have gone to low potencies, making greater and greater failures, to the shame of the tutor and the science they profess to follow. I expect some in the sound of my voice will be doing this five years from now; this is a warning, stop before you go too far, or you will not feel the fault is your own. You will think you were hypnotized and led into false ways. If you neglect making a careful examination the patient will be the first sufferer, but in the end you yourself will suffer from it, and homoeopathy also. The questions themselves that Hahnemann gives are not important, but they are suggestive and will lead you in a certain direction. Question the patient, then the friends, and observe for yourself; if you do not obtain enough to prescribe on, go back to particulars. After much experience you will become expert in questioning patients so as to bring out the truth. Store up Materia Medica so as to use it and it will flow out as your language flows. You must put yourself on a level with the form of speech your patients use.

Be sure you have not put any words into your patient's mouth or biased his expression. You want to know all the particulars but without asking about it directly. If you ask a direct question, you must not put the symptom in the record, for ninety-nine times out of a hundred the patient will answer by 'Yes' or 'No.' If the patient's answer is 'Yes' or 'No,' your question was badly formed. If a question brings no answer let it alone, for he does not know or has not noticed. Questions giving a choice of answers are defective. Ascertain the precise part of the body the pain was in and the character of the pain, etc. In investigating a case there are many things to learn, the length of the attack, appearance of the discharge if it be a case of vomiting, its character, the time of day, etc., etc. Every student should go over these questions framing collateral questions, and practicing case-taking. Leave the patient in freedom always.

Do not put any words into his mouth. Never allow yourself to hurry a patient; get into a fixed habit of examination, then it will stay with you. It is only when you sustain the sharpest kind of work that you can keep your reputation and fulfill your highest use. Say as little as you can, but keep the patient talking and keep him talking close to the line. 1f he will only talk, you can find out symptoms in general and particular. If he goes off, bring him back to the line quietly and without disturbing him. There is not much trouble in private practice. There you will do a better average of work.

All sleep symptoms are important, they are so closely related to the mind, the transfer from sleep to waking, from cerebrum to cerebellum, is important. Old pathologists were unable to account for difficult breathing during sleep. The cerebrum rules respiration during sleep. To know the functions of the white matter and gray matter is important. A rational knowledge of anatomy is important. No homoeopath ever discouraged the true study of anatomy and physiology. It is important not only to know the superficial but the real, profound character, to enable you to recognize one symptom-image from another.

Study this paragraph carefully and meditate upon it. If you do not form habits now, you will not form practice hereafter. You have no regular course and will get into habits you cannot break up.

Classroom Notes

Examination of the Patient

What we are about to consider is, a plan for faithful and careful examination of the case. It is our purpose to cure the case, and it is necessary for this purpose, to bring the patient's symptoms in the very best possible way before the mind. This is a long and a tedious study, and there are many difficulties in the way. One can go about the examination of a patient as follows:

1.   The record can be arranged by dividing the page into three columns. The first contains the dates and prescriptions, the second is for emphatic symptoms, while the third one is for modalities.

2.   Always leave the patient in freedom. Do not put words in his mouth. Say as little as you can, but keep the patient talking and keep him close to line.

3.   Get into a fixed habit of examination then it will stay with you.

4.   After the patient has detailed his sufferings, then proceed to make enquiries. Question the patient, then his friends, and observe for yourself if you do not obtain enough to prescribe then go back to the particulars.

5.   After much experience you will become expert in questioning patients so as to bring out the truth.

6.   If you neglect making a careful physical examination the patient will be the first sufferer, but in the end both you and system will suffer from it.

7.   No Homeopath ever discouraged the true study of anatomy and physiology. It is important not only to know the superficial but the study of real and profound character, to be able to recognize one symptom image from another.

Other Hints and Suggestions:

1.   Mentals are more important.

2.   Sleep symptoms are important.

3.   Menstrual symptoms are important.

4.   The flash of the eye is important, it will tell things that cannot be told by the nurse.

5.   It is important for the physician to know the value of the expression.

6.   The symptoms that arise after the administration of powerful medicine are not indicative of a remedy. (**Drugging is only a master of changing the symptoms and masking the case.**)

7.   Sometimes (mostly in over drugged case), we have to wait a considerable time until the symptoms reveal themselves and express the nature of the sickness.

8.   Very often we have to antidote the over drugged patient.

9.   Then we can take up the thread and get back to the remedy

that was clearly indicated years ago. If the remedy was indicated then but not given, then give the remedy now (Provided the case is not over drugged in such cases you first antidote the drugs and then give the indicated remedy).

10. Remember circumstances of a man's life govern his actions and reactions, symptoms and the development of symptoms. All such circumstances ought to be examined, which sustain or give rise to disease so by their removal cure may be facilitated.

11. Use a keynote to examine the remedy to see if it has all other symptom that patient has.

12. Never prescribe for any two conditions, unless they are complicated. Only Chronic diseases can be complicated with each other. An Acute disease is never complicated with the Chronic. The Acute suppresses the Chronic and they never become Complex.

13. In a complicated case if you are to attempt to prescribe a remedy that has both these groups you would fail to cure. Select the worst one, and entirely ignore the other one. [It is bad policy to give one remedy for one and another for the other] Single out the worst one and cover it carefully with a remedy, and you will find it to disappear and the other one comes on, just as if the patient has not had a remedy at all.

14. Now do not be in a hurry about removing the second disease.

15. You will find that after one has been removed the patient will improve, and the one that has remained will become more and more apparent from day to day, then you prescribe for it.

16. In case of acute on chronic condition or in sequel of acute disease, prescribe first for the acute attack and the symptoms that belong to it. Once the acute attack has settled down, prescribe proper anti-miasmatic remedy.

17. A great deal depends upon the physician's ability to per-

ceive miasma and what symptoms constitute it.

18. Get all the symptoms first and then commence your analysis in relation to remedies. Keep out of the mind while examining a case, some other case that appears to be similar and the remedies that have treated, it in past.

19. The physician must be possessed of an uncommon share of circumspection and tact, knowledge of human heart, prudence and patience, to be able to form a true and complete image of the disease in all its detail and to put patient at ease. Remember the most impatient hypochondriac never invents sufferings and symptoms that are void of foundation. Truth can be known by giving such a patient only placebo and see weather the symptom are consistent or not [if symptoms are not consistent then think hysteria].

20. The Homeopathic physician must be acquainted with the signs and symptoms of human diseases. Different diseases are only a change in combination of those symptoms in manner and representation. There is order, perfect order, in every sickness that presents itself. It rests with the physician to find that order.

LECTURE XXIV

The Examination of the Patient (Continued)

THE examination must be continued with due respect to the nature of the sickness and with due respect to the nature of the Materia Medica. Some symptoms have reference to pathology and diagnosis, while others have reference only to the Materia Medica, and symptoms must be constantly weighed in the mind in order to establish their grade whether common or peculiar. If all are found to be common symptoms, the Materia Medica is left out. Either the examination has not been made with respect to the Materia Medica, or the symptoms are not there at all. It makes no difference as far as cure is concerned; it matters not whether they are not present in the case or whether the doctor has not found them, the key to the prescription is not present. But if the image is round and full and complete, there are symptoms with regard to pathology, diagnosis, prognosis and Materia Medica. It will be proper later to talk of incurable diseases, pathognomic symptoms, obscure cases, Materia Medica symptoms, etc.

When the physician comes to look over the record after an examination to get the image to classify and arrange it, he will find what is peculiar, and those symptoms that are most general, and those that are but common. These three grades appear in every complete case, and in every complete proving of a remedy.

Homoeopathic study and observation will enable one to pick out these grades at a glance. Every case has common symptoms, but peculiar symptoms may be absent and you must not expect to cure when peculiar symptoms are absent. Homoeopathy is applicable in every curable case, but the great thing is to know how to apply it. The physician must sit in judgment upon the symptoms and determine whether they are peculiar or common. If the patient's discourse is incoherent, the question arises is he intoxicated or delirious, or is there breaking down of the brain and insanity? The flash of the eye is important; it will tell things that cannot be told by the nurse.

It is important for the physician to know the value of expressions. When the patient stares with glassy eye, is he injured about the head, is he suffering from shock, intoxication or typhoid fever or some disease in which the mind is stunned? The physician immediately proceeds to ask, "How long has the patient been in bed?" If the character is above reproach, he will not suspect intoxication; if the patient has been sick for many days with fever, tongue coated, abdomen sensitive, etc., he is fully entered upon the course of typhoid fever. The physician must know immediately upon entering the room what the state of the patient resembles: apoplexy, coma, opium poisoning, etc. A physician is supposed to set his mind to work instantly, to ascertain the condition of the patient and what relation the symptoms maintain to the Materia Medica. If an opium poisoning there must be selected an antidote; if apoplexy, a careful taking of the symptoms in relation to the cerebral clot to prevent inflammation and symptoms relative to that state, and relative to the remedy. The patient may be intoxicated and have apoplexy at the same time. There is no symptom in the sick room without its value, especially in acute and serious cases. Children are sometimes found in a sound sleep and cannot be aroused; the mother says the child has worms and gives Cina, for Cina has all these symptoms of stupor, difficulty in arousing, falling back to sleep. But the child fails, going into coma, the nose flaps, the chest heaves, the brow is wrinkled, there is rattling in the chest, showing the child is going into cerebral congestion. The physician now must examine on every side of the case to find the nature, to know what to expect. He who neglects this is not a true homoeopathic physician; a mere superficial application of homeopathy is not sufficient. After all the symptoms are written out, the physician must study the character of the fever, whether it is intermittent, continued or has come on in one sudden attack; he must know sufficient of the symptoms to judge of all these. You will learn so much about the purport and the aspect of every motion of the human being that you will place less and less reliance on diagnostic symptoms as diagnostic symptoms, and learn more the value of symptoms as symptoms. You will be astonished to find how expert you will become about diagnosis and prognosis by studying the symptoms. You can learn something from every case you have mind; but by a process of rapid exclusion, you say it is not into mind; but by a process of rapid exclusion, you say it is not cholera, not haemorrhage, etc., and latterly you come to the cause of this aspect. You can tell when it is time for cardiac compensation to be broken in Bright's disease; a peculiar tremulous wave that belongs to the muscles of the face and neck, a tremulous jerk of the tongue, putting about half way; the pale, cold, semi-transparent skin with cold sweat. It is important to know instantly what the cause is, for the treatment will be different, but remember that it is nothing that you need to name that makes it important.

All these symptoms have respect to remedy and to diagnostic conditions. So far as there is a morbid anatomy which can account for symptoms, so much less are those symptoms worth, as indicating a remedy; if you had no other than such symptoms, you could find no remedy.

Among the many things that interfere with the examination of the patient the most important is the taking of medicines, or having done something, no matter what it is, that has been capable of changing the symptoms. Very commonly, the patient will present himself in the doctor's office, and after giving a long array of symptoms will relate a dose of Quinine, and he thinks he is no better, and now he applies to you for relief. In acute diseases this is very bad and may interfere with finding the homoeopathic remedy. Very often the general state collectively both drug and disease symptoms, in a very acute condition must be prescribed for, but in chronic disease the plan is different. The symptoms that arise after the taking of a dose of powerful medicine are not indicative of a remedy, they are confusing, they present no true image of the disease and hence the physician has nothing to do but wait, or at most administer a well-known antidote to the drug taken. Sometimes he must wait a considerable time until the symptoms reveal themselves and express the nature of the sickness. It is just as bad where the physician himself is a bungler as it is where the patient has taken the drugs. The confusion arising from bad prescribing is just the same as that produced by the patient's drugging. There are physicians going about who will mix up their cases and continue to prescribe for their own drug symptoms, and who never have any idea of waiting for the true image of the disease to develop itself. Drugging is only a matter of changing symptoms and masking the case. Anything that will effect a change in the symptoms, the taking of drugs, or drinking too much wine or drinking toddy, or great exposure, will mask the case, and this mask must wear away before the intelligent physician can make a cure. The whole aim of the physician is to secure the language of nature. If it has been masked by medicines, it cannot be secured. Any meddling will so affect the aspect of the case that the physician cannot prescribe, and the physician who does this meddling must inevitably be driven into bad methods or into allopathy. I have looked over the work of bad prescribers and have wondered what on earth they could see in homoeopathy to attract them; they do not cure folks. They have no cures to present. The patients cannot well be satisfied by these things. It is true that once in a while a strong, vigorous, robust patient, when he gets a homoeopathic remedy, will go on getting well through a mess of symptom changing and drugging, so that in spite of this meddlesome practice he will recover. The physician in that case, knows not what remedy to attribute to it, for he has given a great many. But only the most vigorous constitution will stand such homoeopathic villainy, go on and get well in spite of their indulgence in wine, in eating, etc.; it is wonderful what their own powers will do in throwing off disease.

In ordinary cases, however, we see no such things; confusion is brought about at once if the physician administer another medicine in place of administering placebo. At times a patient will present himself, and you will be able to get a true image of the sickness by ascertaining all the things that occurred up to a given date. "'Upon that date," he says, "I took some medicine, and most of my symptoms subsided." They lead to another image from which you can gather nothing; a scattering has taken place. The symptoms may cover page upon page, and yet what remedy do you see? None at all; it looks as if a number of provings of drugs had been mixed up all together, intermingling symptoms here and there without any distinctness. No individualization is possible. Now up to that date the symptoms you gathered may be just all that is necessary. Up to that date the symptoms present the image of a remedy which, if administered, may yet act, though sometimes it will fail at first because of the confusion, but after waiting a little it will act. After the administration of a remedy prescribed upon symptoms in the past I have known the remedy many times to go on acting. Again I have known that remedy to fail entirely. In such a case, wait awhile and then order will begin to come and that remedy which was indicated previous to the drugging will act. Suppose a physician comes to you and says, "Up to a certain date I was able to hold this patient's symptoms in order with Thuja occidentalis; but then the symptoms seemed to change and I gave such and such medicines, and have never seen such good results in prescribing as I did up to that period." You must give him Thuja occidentalis again, and in this way take up the thread where it was lost. Examine the image of the case where the order was lost; because that is where the image must be found. "On the contrary, the symptoms and the inconveniences which exhibited themselves previous to the use of the medicines, or several days after their discontinuance, give the true fundamental notion of the original form of the malady."

This is the idea, get the original form of the malady. To do this, at times we have to trace through a mass of difficulties and conditions to get back to the original form of the trouble, but you must get there because you will see that in the beginning this malady, in accordance with all laws of Divine Providence, must have conformed to some remedy that had been created for its cure. The symptoms at that time stood out indicating this medicine, but since then there has been nothing but confusion, nothing that can be tied to, nothing that can be examined; it appears to have no relation to anything. Very often we can take up the thread and get back to the remedy that was clearly indicated, even twenty years before. If that remedy was indicated then, and was not given, the cure that was possible by that remedy or a similar one is the only thing to be considered; that is the only remedy in the case. Since that time the patient has been in continued turmoil from the action of drugs. Because it was twenty years ago there is no reason that you should not think of that drug. The patient's disease has not been cured, it has only been changed and modified; but it is the same patient, and the same sickness and requires the same medicine. If the disease has been complicated by drugs, however, you cannot always get the action of that medicine which the patient needs for the disease *per se*, but after the drugs have been antidoted you will have to give that very medicine that you figured out and he will be cured.

It is necessary also to observe the changes all along the line of progress, to know the disease at its beginnings, its earlier manifestations, its symptoms and its endings. You find, say, most violent neuralgic pains along the course of nerves in an adult patient, and for these you administer remedies until you are tired and get only temporary relief; but you discover that in his childhood he had an eczema, and you will find it look like *Mezereum*, and see its violent neuralgias are similar to those of your patient. The administration of *Mezereum* cures this neuralgia and brings back the eruption that he had in his babyhood, and he goes on to recovery. Without getting that view of the old scald head, you would not have thought of *Mezereum*.

Or, instead of *Mezereum*, *Sepia officinalis* may have had the likeness of that scald head, and he may now have the most striking and characteristic symptoms of *Sepia*; for behold the little things that have been put into such a turmoil by a bad drugging are under *Sepia*, and you put your patient on *Sepia*, and these last appearing symptoms go first and the eruption comes back upon the head and behind the ears, and *Sepia* has cured him. When these things are seen one after another in everyday practice the physician must begin to wonder if there is not some truth in it all. And as sure as you live, if you practice faithfully, carefully studying your cases at great length, gathering in everything that was in the beginning, your cures will be so striking that the multitude will come to you to be healed. You cannot place too much importance upon the masking of a patient's symptoms by medicines, by improper repetitions and by dosing carelessly.

§ 94. "On inquiry into a state of chronic disease it is required to weigh the particular circumstances in which the patient may be placed in regard to ordinary occupation, mode of life and domestic situation," etc. Almost everything in life is circumstantial. All of the activities of life are circumstantial, *i.e.*, there are no activities that are not governed by circumstance. There is no business that is not governed by circumstance. The circumstances of a man's life govern his actions and reactions, symptoms and the development of symptoms. The body is associated with circumstances, every function is related to circumstance, and we may say all the natural functions of life are connected with circumstances. Without these we would have nothing to prescribe upon, we would have nothing to ascertain images by, we would have nothing to form the symptoms, hence the circumstances of life and habit must be studied with a view to going into the slightest particulars. To illustrate that more particularly, and to bring it down to a practical basis, we may say that the examination of every woman relates to her eating, her stool, her menstruation, her bathing, her dress, because these are the things natural to her. These are the circumstances in which her symptoms may come or may not come.

Until the woman is educated to it she does not understand, "What do you mean, Doctor?" she says. Then I may say, "You have given me these symptoms; you say you have headache, stomachache, etc. Now will you proceed to relate to me under what circumstances this headache appears, how it is affected by your changes in dress, by the changes in weather, how it is affected before, during or after your monthly indisposition and so on," Now, these are the natural circumstances.

In addition to these another group of circumstances comes up, a group of circumstances somewhat different, in relation to ordinary occupation. Every person will have circumstances more particular than those in general. Occupation will make changes in the circumstances of young women. She may be standing upon the floor of Wanamaker's store all day, and this has produced a condition of prolapsus; or she may lead a sedentary life at her work as seamstress, or she may be at some other occupation, the circumstance of which will develop her psoric manifestations. Modes of life mean a great many different things. They come in as supernumeraries over and above the natural conditions and circumstances of life. The natural functions and circumstances of life have to be considered in relation to the mode of life. The mode of life comes in as, the exciting cause of disease, whereby psora which is in the economy is developed in a certain peculiar direction.

The domestic is often the cause of trouble in the woman; there may be marriage to a man who is intemperate with her sexually; she may have a domestic situation that cannot be cured, and it must be examined as to its permanency and the prospect of removing it. Things that cannot be removed will develop psora, in a peculiar direction. "All these circumstances ought to be examined to discover if there is anything that could give birth to and keep up the disease, so that by its removal the cure may be facilitated."

LECTURE XXV

The Examination of the Patient (Continued)

§ 92. THE patients generally call attention to the commonest things, while it is the strange and peculiar things that guide to a remedy. The symptoms most covered up from the observation of the physician are often the things guiding to the remedy, but finally they leak out in some way. The symptom is of such a character that the patient says of it, "I have always had it and did not suppose that had anything to do with my disease." When asked, "Why did you not tell me that before?" she says, "I did not suppose that amounted to anything, it is so trivial." The physician often hazards a remedy. He feels he must make a prescription, but has no reasonable grounds for thinking he has found the remedy because the patient's story has been so confusing, and the symptoms that he has obtained are so common and ordinary, such as all remedies possess. With such a foundation he cannot have any assurance that he has the remedy, and, although he may have hazarded several remedies in the case, the patient comes back uncured, month after month, and year after year. These symptoms that are withheld and seem to be so obscure, and so difficult to obtain, are the very ones that the patient thinks do not amount to anything. What seems to him to be the little symptoms are very often characteristic of the disease, and necessary for the choice of the remedy. Let me illustrate it. A patient comes along with a pallid face, a rather sickly countenance, tired and weary, subject to headaches, disorders of the bladder and disturbances of digestion; and in spite of all your questioning, you fail to get anything that is peculiar. You set the patient to thinking and to writing down symptoms, and she comes back month after month and give her *Sulphur, Lycopodium* and a good many medicines. You can sometimes find out whether she is a chilly or hot-blooded patient, and thus you can get a little closer among the common remedies; but the patient says one day, "Doctor, it seems strange that urine smells so queer, it smells like that of a horse." Now at once you know that is *Nitricum acidum.* "How long have you had this?" "Oh, I have always had it, I did not think it amounted to anything." If you examine the common things belonging to *Nitricum acidum* you will find that it possesses all the features of the case.

This is how a guiding symptom can be used. *Nitricum acidum* has a keynote "urine smelling strong like that of a horse;" but if you should give it upon that alone and the general symptoms were not there, you would probably remove the particular symptoms only, and they would come back after a while. Use a keynote to examine the remedy to see if it has all the other symptoms that the patient has. What I have described to you is a hypothetical case. In a busy day you will have several of these cases that you have been working at for months, and the patients have spent a lot of money to no account. You might just as well have given *Sac. lac.* until you found the right remedy. You can hardly say, why did I not see the remedy before, because it was not possible to see it. You can only go over a case and say, why did I not ask her if there was any odor to the urine, and if so, what it was like. I have had this very symptom come out when I have asked a dozen times about the smell of the urine, and they did not know, and yet would say afterwards their urine smelled like a horse's urine, and they knew it all the time. "On the other hand, the patients are so accustomed to their long sufferings that they pay little or no attention to the lesser symptoms which are often characteristic of the disease and decisive in regard to the choice of a remedy."

Of course the trouble that we have to contend with in ascertaining symptoms from patients could be drawn out to great length. You might suppose that it would be the educated class that would tell their symptoms best, but you will find the ignorant class often do better, they are simpler; they do not disguise the symptoms; they come out and tell the little details in a better way, in a way that conforms to the language of our remedies. Our remedies have been recorded in simple language to a great extent, and this simple language is often better observed by the simple-minded, uncultivated people than among the aristocrats. People who have plenty of means and much education are more excitable, they have more fear and they have tried a great many doctors. Any physician who has a reputation is consulted for a chronic disease; and the patient who has plenty of money goes around amongst the doctors, and when he comes to tell his symptoms he tells them in the technicalities of his numerous physicians, so that when he has finished his story nothing has been gained. Only gradually can the physician lead him back into a language simple enough to describe the sufferings. They who have been sick long with their chronic ailments and have become somewhat hypochondriac will go through with this list of their diseases. They have paid lots of money, and have lots of names, and they are loaded with drugs. The physician must deal very carefully with these slippery people, because if they are irritated they will run off.

§ 96. There is another kind of patient spoken of here, those that "depict their sufferings in lively colors, and make use of exaggerated terms to induce the physician to relieve them promptly." This is especially characteristics of the native Irish as a class. You will find that they will exaggerate their symptoms, really and sincerely believing that the doctor will give them stronger medicine if they are very sick and will pay more attention to them; and if they do not exaggerate violently, probably he will turn them off with a simple remedy. Then we have the exaggeration of symptoms by sensitive people. It is an insane habit, such as belong to hysteria. The physician will be helpless in the hands of these exaggerators, because homoeopathy consists in securing the whole truth and nothing but the truth; it is just as detrimental to get too much as to get too little. Any coloring that is expressed, whether by the patient or by the physician, will result in failure. It is true that this tendency to exaggeration must be considered as a symptom. When you have found a patient to exaggerate a few symptoms into a large number, you can simply mention in your note "tendency to exaggerate symptoms," which is covered by some of our remedies. Such a state is misleading, for you do not know what symptoms the patient has and what the patient has not. You may rest assured that no patient without symptoms would consult a physicians; the patient would not be likely to manufacture the entire sickness; the fact that she has a desire to present herself to the physician and has a desire to exaggerate her symptoms and sufferings is in itself a disease, because no well person would do that. Hence this must be considered; perhaps it is the first and only element that can be considered of that which such patients give out. This exaggeration must be measured with discretion and wisdom. "Even the most impatient hypochrondriac never invents sufferings and symptoms that are void of foundation, and the truth of this is easily ascertained by comparing the complaints he utters at different intervals while the physician gives him nothing at least that is medicinal:" Hahnemann's plan would he to give no medicine and to compare the symptoms that the patient gives from time to time. The patient cannot memorize these various symptoms that he has gathered from other sources, but by watching and comparing from time to time, letting the examination be far enough apart for him to forget, the physician can accept those things that he repeats. The young physician will be misguided by these cases until he has had sufficient experience with disease to know something about the nature of symptoms that ought to appear.

Another obstacle we have in the examination of the case is laziness; the patient is too lazy to write down the symptoms when they appear, and too indolent and forgetful to remember them in the presence of the physician. The symptoms do not come up in his mind when he is in the presence of the doctor, and he is too indolent to write these symptoms down when he feels them at home. When a patient does not relate symptoms well he should be instructed to write down his symptoms when they occur, and if he will not do that his physician should insist upon it, or refuse to prescribe for him. It is often quite an important thing to get the patient to write down the symptoms in memorandum form as they occur. Not to write at night what has occurred during the day, but to run instantly and put the symptom down in simple language, describing the sensation, and location, and the time of day of its coming and going, and the modalities. Indolence then and forgetfulness become obstacles to the gathering of the symptoms.

Now, in the present day, there has crept upon the face of the earth such a state of false modesty and such a lack of innocence upon the whole human race that this false modesty and shame will prevent patients from telling the truth. Patients will deny having had gonorrhoea, or having been exposed to circumstances that were similar. If the whole human race had lived in innocence up to the present day our women would come to the physician with frankness and talk in perfect freedom concerning the menstrual flow, concerning even the sexual functions, concerning things of the will and of the intelligence. But as a matter of fact it is not so, it is with difficulty that the physicians can draw out these symptoms through mistaken modesty. When a patient consults a physician, the question of modesty should be laid aside. You will find that the most innocent in mind are those that are the most easy to lay it aside, when it is not a question of modesty, but of telling the whole truth and nothing but the truth. If it be a wife, everything that is in relation to herself and husband that is abnormal should be told, and then the physician would have little to ask beyond listening to the truth. I look back over a number of people, especially among women, when seemed to be so much embarrassed upon first coming into my presence and having to talk about their symptoms that they forget everything, and it was only by considerable waiting that they became free and frank and open with me. Sometimes it is a difficult matter for the physician to put a patient at ease; it is a thing that must be studied and considered in order to be able to say something to put a bashful patient at ease; this is quite an accomplishment with a doctor.

The physician must be possessed of an uncommon share of circumspection and tact, a knowledge of the human heart, prudence and patience, to be enabled to form to himself a true and complete image of the disease in all its details. He must live the life of the neighbour, and be known as a man of honour, as a man who may be believed and respected, as a candid man. Hahnemann says carelessness, laziness and levity will prevent the physician from going into such a state of homoeopathy as will enable him to grasp the Materia Medica or to be conversant with his science. If he has such a reputation he will not command the respect of the people of the neighbourhood, and this will prevent him from getting the image of the sickness upon paper. Hahnemann had a wonderful knowledge of the human heart, and this is an important thing; a knowledge of the human heart, a knowledge of the things that are in man.

It would seem that there are a good many men in the community without the slightest knowledge of the human heart. They have never given any inspection to their own interiors, their heart or impulses, but have gone on wildly. To know the human heart well is largely to examine into oneself and ascertain what one's own impulses are, what one is compelled to do under varying circumstances, what impulses one has to control in oneself in order to become a man. If a man has carried out his heart's desires without any self-control he is a man unworthy of respect. If he has on the other hand controlled those impulses, he has become a man worthy of respect. In time the physician who does this will become so well acquainted with the human heart that he has sympathy and knows what constitutes the language of the affections.

LECTURE XXVI

The Examination of the Patient (Continued)

IT is important to avoid getting confused by two disease images that may exist in the body at the same time. A chronic patient, for instance, may be suffering from an acute disease and the physician on being called may think that it is necessary to take the totality of the symptoms; but if he should do that in an acute disease, mixing both chronic and acute symptoms together, he will become confused and will not find the right remedy. The two things must be separated. The group of symptoms that constitutes the image and appearance of the acute miasm must now be prescribed for. The chronic symptoms will not, of course, be present when the acute miasm is running, because the latter suppresses or suspends the chronic symptoms, but the diligent physician, not knowing this is so, might wrongly gather together all the symptoms that the patient has had in a life time. Again, on the other hand, in gathering together the chronic symptoms for a prescription it is sufficient to mention merely that the patient has had typhoid or measles or other acute miasms. Such diseases are not a part of the chronic miasm. The symptoms of the acute attack were separate and by themselves.

You must realize that the effort to prescribe for two distinct miasms will result in error. If you practice in the western part of this country you will often get confused cases, a sample of which would be about as follows: A patient has been suffering from intermittent fever, and has been treated with medicines, Quinine, Arsenic and low potencies of this and that drug, until the case has been complicated. You learn that the symptoms now are different from what they were in the beginning, that there has been a transformation scene. You prescribe for them as they are now, regarding it as a species of malaria; you prescribe for them with a view to antidoting all the drugs that he has had, and your remedy brings about a surprise; it opens out the case in a wonderful manner. The patient up to this time was unable to give you anything descriptive of the original state of his malaria, but he comes back in the course of a week or two and says: "Doctor, I am now as I was in the beginning:' "Well, what are your symptoms now?" And you will find out that one evening he has a 5 o'clock chill with its accompanying symptoms that last him a good portion of the night, and then he has a well day, and then next forenoon he has an 11 o'clock chill and then a well day. If you examine each one of these states, you will find that the two chills begin in a different place, and the heat of each begins in a different place, and the symptoms of the two attacks are totally different. Such a thing will seem unlikely to one who has never seen it, but one who has lived in the west and practiced accurately will see such things, unknown to those who have practiced what is called Quinine Homoeopathy. A correct prescription will disentangle these two malarial miasms and show that two exist in the body at the same time, each having conditions quite different from the other. These two can co-exist and have their own times and expressions without interfering with each other to any great extent. The big doses of Quinine will complicate them and cause a general clouding of things, so helterskelter and disorderly that nobody can tell anything about it.

If in such a case you were to attempt to prescribe a remedy that had both these groups you would fail to cure. Select the worst one, and let the other one alone, entirely ignoring it. It is a bad policy to give one remedy for one and another for the other. Single out the worst one and cover it carefully with a remedy, and you will find it disappear and the other one comes on, just as if the patient had not a remedy at all.

Now do not be in too great a hurry about removing the second one. You will find that after one has been removed the patient will improve, and the one that has remained will become more and more apparent from day to day; then prescribe for it.

This illustrates the doctrine of not prescribing for an acute and chronic trouble together. Never prescribe for any two conditions, unless they be complicated. Only chronic diseases can be complicated with each other. The acute is never complicated with the chronic; the acute suppresses the chronic and they never become complex. Of course, the allopaths will tell you about the sequelae of measles, scarlet fever, etc., but they know nothing about it, and their pathology teaches them nothing which is true concerning it. That which comes out after all self-limiting diseases have run their course is not due to the disease itself; the sequelae of measles are not due to measles, the sequelae of scarlet fever are not due to scarlet fever, but to a prior state of the patient. A psoric disorder may come after scarlet fever or measles, and must be treated as psora.

These sequelae, regardless of the disease which stirs them up, are psoric and crop out at the weakest time, which is the convalescent period. The better the acute disease is treated, the less likely there are to be any sequelae. If measles and scarlet fever are treated properly we have very little trouble afterwards. Sequelae should always be charged up to a great extent to the physician. Of course, you will find now and then some constitutions extremely psoric; almost in a condition of advanced decay, and for malignant scarlet fever in such a patient it is difficult to find a proper remedy, and then the very best physician in the world may make a mistake; yet with good treatment in ordinary cases you should not expect sequelae, such as sore eyes, running ears, etc.

It is of the greatest importance in such cases to be able to separate and distinguish one thing from another, so that you may know what you are prescribing for. You cannot prescribe an antipsoric in order to prevent sequelae following scarlet fever while the scarlet fever prevails. Prescribe first for the acute attack, and the symptoms that belong to it. It is well, however, for the physician to know all the symptoms that the patient has of a chronic character, that he may know what to expect, that he may look at the close of the acute attack for the coming out of the old manifestations of psora, although often an entirely new group of symptoms will appear. When at the close of scarlet fever troubles come about the ears or dropsical conditions come on; these are not a part of the scarlet fever itself, but of the state of the economy. The dropsical condition, or acute Bright's disease, must be associated with the psoric state and the symptoms then will lead you to a constitutional remedy. If you have in view simply the Bright's disease, you will make a mistake. You will fall into prescribing for ultimates if you have but the name of the trouble in mind, for instance giving *Apis,* which the books say, is a wonderful remedy for Bright's disease, following scarlet fever.

It is a great mistake for anyone to fit remedies for complaints or states. It is a fatal error for the physician to go on the bedside of a patient with the feeling in his mind that he has had cases similar to this one, and thinking thus: "In the last case I had I gave so and so, therefore I will give it to this one." The physician must get such things entirely out of his mind. It is a common feature among occulists who profess to be homoeopaths to say: "I cured such and such a case with such and such a remedy. I will now give this patient the same remedy." I have many times met physicians in consultations who said: "I have another patient, Mr. Z or Mr. X, who had a similar state of affairs, just such a disease as this, and I gave him so and so; but it does not work in this case."

§ 100. "With regard to a search after the totality of the symptoms in epidemic and sporadic cases, it is wholly indifferent whether anything similar ever existed before in the world or not, under any name whatever." Keep that in your mind, underscore it half a dozen times with red ink, paint it on the wall, put all index finger to it. One of the most important things is to keep out of the mind, in an examination of the case, some other case that has appeared to be similar. If this is not done the mind will be prejudiced in spite of your best endeavors. I have to fight that with every fresh case I come to. I have to labour to keep myself from thinking about things I have cured like that before, because it would prejudice my mind.

The purpose of all this is that you will go away and examine the patient with an unprejudiced mind, that you will consider only the case before you, that you will have nothing in mind that will distract your attention, that you may not think of things that preceded it and find out from among them a remedy while examining the patient. If you are biased in your judgment and examine the patient towards a certain remedy, in many instances this will prove to be fatal. Have no remedy in mind until you have everything that you can get on paper. Have it all written down carefully and then if, upon examining it in relation to remedies, you are unable to distinguish between three or four, you can go back and re-examine the patient with reference to those three or four remedies.

That is the only possible time you try to fit a remedy, or image of a remedy, while examining a patient. Get all the symptoms first and then commence your analysis in relation to remedies. The analysis of a sickness is for the purpose of gathering together that about it which is peculiar, for the peculiar thing relate to remedies. Sicknesses have in them that which is peculiar, strange and rare, and the things in sickness that may be wondered at are things to be compared with those in the remedy that are peculiar. Now in order to see that which is wonderful and strange it is necessary for you to have much knowledge of disease and much knowledge of Materia Medica; not so much an extensive knowledge of morbid anatomy, but a knowledge of the symptoms or the language that disease expresses itself in. "In fact, we ought to regard the pure image of each prevailing disease as a thing that is new and unknown, and study the same from its foundation, if we would really exercise the art of healing." A great deal depends upon a physician's ability to perceive what constitutes the miasm. If he is dull of perception he will intermingle symptoms that do not belong together. Hahnemann seems to have had the most wonderful perception, he seemed to see at a glance. Hahnemann was skilful in this respect because he was a hard student of Materia Medica and because he proved his Materia Medica daily. He had examined the remedies carefully, he saw them, he felt them, he realized them. "We ought never to substitute hypothesis in the room of observation, never regard any case as already known." Now we see why it is that it does not make any difference with a physician whether he has seen such diseases before or not. The homoeopathic physician is acquainted with the signs and symptoms of the man, and a different disease is only a change in the combination of them, only a change in their manner, form and representation. There is order, perfect order, in every sickness that presents itself, and it rests with the physician to find that order. The homoeopathic physician need never be taken unawares.

LECTURE XXVII

§ 103, ETC. Record Keeping

YOU should endeavor to have a good knowledge of both the acute and chronic miasms. First of all the image of psora should be studied from all the symptoms that we can gather, and especially from the symptoms that Hahnemann has given, in the *Chronic Diseases*. Next we have to make out a similar anamnesis of syphilis, which can be done from books, from clinics, from observation, and all other possible sources, and then an anamnesis has to be made of sycosis. These are things most general, and will bring before the mind, in one, two or three images, a grand picture of all the chronic diseases of the human race.

Take psora first for that is the very foundation of human sickness. It would appear that the human race is one enormous leper. Now, add to that the state of syphilis and we have a bad matter made worse; then add to that the state of sycosis and we will see the extent of human sickness.

We then have to advance and carefully study each of the acute miasms from the books, from observation, and from every source of information, carefully arranging it on paper so that it can appear before the mind as an image. Smallpox has few features and it can be made to appear as an image before the mind, and so with all the acute miasms, infectious diseases, cholera, yellow fever, etc., the diseases that have here-to-before appeared in epidemic or endemic form. These have all to appear before the mind as images. It may be said of them that they are all true diseases seen by the examination of the totality of the symptoms. No physician can know too much about the image of a given sickness, studied from the symptomatology, and this is the best information that can be obtained. Now-a-days patients are not permitted to tell their story in the language of nature. The physician says, "I do not want to hear that." Talk on the part of the patient interferes with his prescription writing. There is no writing down of the case.

Now take, for instance, one of the clinics here. How would you remember from day to day, and from week to week, what had been given to each patient? There is no importance attached to that in the old school. It is simply their object to give the patient a big dose of medicine. It may not have occurred to you that there are several reasons of importance for keeping records, and of constantly referring to them; even the regular clinicians here may not have seen the full importance of it. But suppose a patient that I have been considering for three years is partially cured, and she has done remarkably well, has been restored from an invalid to a good wife and mother, but is not yet cured. Now for some reason she goes into the hands of another homoeopath. What can he do without ascertaining what I have done for her? It is important for the patient when living in the same town to be faithful and true to the physician who has done her the most good. A conscientious physician will not feel like taking another doctor's practice in that way. I am not so conceited that I should feel like taking up the work of another doctor who is able to do good work. Men who think more of getting money than anything else will jump in and prescribe for your patients.

"The physician ought ever after to have this image before the eyes to serve as a basis to the treatment, especially where the disease is chronic." Without records, you are at sea without compass or rudder. With a record, Hahnemann says, "He can then study it in all its parts, and draw from it the characteristic marks," that is, you have the nature of the disease continuously in mind. When the image of the disease has passed from mind its very nature is gone.

Here a point comes in you must know about. After your first prescription has been made, you may have an aggravation. It is well to know the date of this, and about how long it lasted, and to keep watch of it. If no change has occurred the same image may continue to appear before the mind, but if changes have occurred and are continuously appearing in the symptoms you will readily see that no medicine can be administered. The symptoms that come and go could not guide anybody as to what to do. Now a commotion has taken place, you cannot prescribe while this commotion is going on, the symptoms are changing place, they are coming and going, for perhaps one to three weeks after that prescription. You have to watch and wait. Notice when the symptoms begin to roll into order; then another dose of medicine is needed.

These things take place only after the administration of a remedy that was pretty high, high enough to take hold, and the case falls into order only when the patient needs another dose.

Suppose a patient has been sick three to four years with a train of symptoms, and on the way to visit you from a long distance; the patient is taken worse, and a homoeopathic physician is called in. The patient gets a dose of medicine and improves wonderfully, now what are you going to do? You do not know what it was and you write to the physician, but he has forgotten what it was. What a confusing state that is, is it not? Well, that is just the state you would be in without your records.

There is, I have been led to feel, too great carelessness often among our best men in transferring cases from one town to another, from one physician to another. A habit that has existed between another Hahnemannian and myself has been pleasing to us both. When one of his patients has been transferred from his care to my care he has told me what remedy the patient was on, and I in the same way when sending patients to, him have mentioned the remedy the patient was on. It is the duty of the physician to furnish such information when a patient leaves the city to go under the care of another physician. It is the duty of the physician to transfer such a patient to good hands, if there are any good hands to transfer him to.

This subject is preliminary to the observation of § 105, which leads to the second step of practical homoeopathy.

Classroom Notes

Record Keeping

Record keeping is a matter of individual choice. Don't be compelled to follow any scheme.

Do keep a record of every case.

LECTURE XXVIII

§ 105, Etc. The Study of Provings

IT may be well for you to review thoroughly the first portion of the study of the *Organon*, containing the doctrines in general that may be hereafter found to be useful in the application of homoeopathy, including the oldest established rules and principles. The first step may be called theoretical homoeopathy, or the principles of homoeopathy after which we take up the homoeopathic method of studying sickness. In this way we have found that the study of sickness in our school is entirely different from the study of sickness under the old school. But up to this time the doctrines have not exhibited their purpose; we only get their purpose when we come to the third step, which deals with the use of Materia Medica. We have seen that we must study sickness by gathering the symptoms of sick patients, relying upon the symptoms as the language of nature, and that the totality of the symptoms constitutes the nature and quality and all there is that is to be known of the disease.

The subject we will now take up and consider is, how to acquire a knowledge of the instruments that we shall make use of in combating human sickness. We know very well that in the old school there is no plan laid down for acquiring a knowledge of medicines except by experimenting with them upon the sick. This Hahnemann condemns as dangerous, because it subjects human sufferers to hardship and because of its uncertainty. Though this system has existed for many hundreds of years, it has never revealed a principle or method that one can take hold of to help in curing the sickness of the human family. His experiments in drug proving were made before he studied diseases. In other words, Hahnemann built the Materia Medica and then took up the plan of examining the patient to see what remedy the sickness looked like. Whereas now, after homoeopathy has been established, and the Materia Medica has been established, the examination of the patient precedes, in a particular case, the examination of the Materia Medica. But for the purpose of study they go hand in hand.

Before Hahnemann could examine the Materia Medica you may say he had to make one, for there was none to examine, there were no provings as yet; we now have the instruments before us to examine, we have the proved remedies. When did the fallacy of old school medicine fully entered Hahnemanns mind; when he became disgusted with its method at the time his children were sick; when he placed himself in the stream of Providence and affirmed his trust that the Lord had not made these little ones to suffer, and then to be made worse from violent medicines; then his mind was in an attitude for discovery. It was a discountenancing of and disgust for the things that were useless, and this brought him to the state of acknowledgment of not knowing and that everything of man's own opinion must be thrown away. It brought him to a state of humility and the acknowledgment of Divine Providence.

The state of humility opens man's mind. You will find so long as man is in a position to trust himself he makes himself a god; he makes himself the infallible; he looks to himself and does not see beyond himself; his mind is then closed. When a man finds out that in himself he is a failure, that is the beginning of knowledge in any circumstance; the very opposite of this closes the mind and turns man away from knowledge.

I have been teaching long enough to observe, and I will tell you some things I have observed. I have observed quite a number of young people turn away from homoeopathy after once confessing it, and professing to practice it, and after seeming able in a certain degree to practice it. I often wondered why it was that after they had made public profession of it they turned away from it, and I found in every instance that it was due to lack of humility. The great mistake comes from turning one's attention into self and relying upon self, with an attention that closes the mind and deprives one of knowledge and prevents clear perception. Man takes himself out of the stream of Providence when he becomes dissatisfied with himself and thinks "now that I have done so many things I have nothing more to study," This is a wrong attitude; for anything like self-conceit will blind a mans eyes, will make him unable to use the means of cure and will prevent his becoming acquainted with the Materia Medica. The homoeopathic physician, as much as the clergyman, ought to keep himself in a state of purity, a state of humility, a state of innocence. So sure as he does not do that he will fall by the wayside. There is nothing that destroys a man so fast in the scientific world as conceit. We see in old-fashioned science men who are puffed up and corpulent with conceit. The scientific men who are in the greatest degree of simplicity are the most wise and the most worthy, and you need not tell me that those who are innocent and simple have not had a tremendous struggle in order to keep self under control and to reach this state of simplicity.

Extensive knowledge makes a man simple, makes him gentle. Extensive knowledge makes a man realize how little he knows, and what a small concern he is. A little knowledge makes a fool of man, and makes him think he knows it all, and the more he forgets of what he has known the bigger man he feels he is. The smaller he feels he is the more he knows, you may rest assured. In order to do this, he must study and keep himself in a state of gravity and in a state of innocence.

In the scientific world we have all those horrible jealousies and feelings of hatred to those who know more than we do. A man who cannot control that and keep that down is not fit to enter the science of homoeopathy. He must be innocent of these things; he must put that aside and be willing to learn of all sources, providing the truth flows from these sources. In this frame of mind, and this frame of mind only, can the physician proceed to examine the Materia Medica.

We have already said that Hahnemann had no Materia Medica to start with. He could not go to books, and read, and meditate, and find remedies in the image of human sickness. He had no such remedies to study, and hence it was necessary to build up the Materia Medica. We can imagine that Hahnemann must have been almost in a state of despair, and inclined to say there is no knowledge upon the earth. He felt in his own mind that we should never know anything about the Materia Medica so long as we perceived its effects only in human sickness, but that a true and pure Materia Medica must be formed by observing the action of medicines upon the healthy human race. Hahnemann did not commence to feed these medicines to others; he took the Peruvian Bark himself, and felt its effects upon himself. He allowed it to manifest its symptoms, and when he had thus proved Peruvian Bark (which we call *China*) it might be then said that the first remedy known to man was discovered, and that the first drug effect was known and that *China* was born! Hahnemann searched the literature of the day to find out what other effects of *China* had been discovered accidentally, and accepted such as were in harmony with what he had discovered. We have already referred to the fact that Hahnemann was able, after proving *China*, to see that in its action it closely resembled the intermittent fevers that had existed through all time; that there was the most abundant relation of similitude between *China* and intermittent fever. Do we wonder, then, that Hahnemann said to himself, can it be possible that the law of cure is the law of similars? Can it be possible that similars are cured by drugs that produce symptoms like unto the sickness? Every drug he proved thereafter established the law more and more, made it appear more certain, and every drug that he proved added one more remedy to the instrument that we call the Materia Medica, until it came to be what we now recognize as Hahnemann's Materia Medica Pura and the Materia Medica of the Chronic Diseases. This work was simply enormous and very thorough, but many additions have been made to it since the time of its publication, and these form the instruments we have to examine.

The best way to study a remedy is to make a proving of it. Suppose we were about to do that; suppose this class were entering upon a proving. Each member of the class would devote, say, a week, in examining carefully all the symptoms that he or she is the victim of, or believes himself or herself to be the victim of, at the present time, and for many months back. Each student then proceeds to write down carefully all these symptoms and places them by themselves. This group of symptoms is recognized as the diseased state of that individual.

A master-prover is decided upon, who will prepare for the proving a substance unknown to the class and to all the provers, known only to himself. He will begin with the first or earliest form of the drug, it may be the tincture, and potentize it to the 30th potency, putting a portion of that potency into a separate vial for each member of the class. The provers do not know what they are taking, and they are requested not to make known to each other their symptoms. When their own original symptoms appear in the proving the effect of the remedy upon anyone of these chronic symptoms is simply noted, whether cured or exaggerated, or whether or not interfered with; but when the symptom occurs in its own natural way, without being increased or diminished, it may be looked upon as one of the natural things of that particular prover, and hence all the natural things of the prover are eliminated. Generally if a remedy takes a marked hold of a prover all the chronic symptoms will subside, but when a proving only takes a partial hold it may only create a few symptoms. These few symptoms, when added to the symptoms that the other provers have felt, will go to make up the chronic effect of the remedy, which may be said to be the effect of the remedy upon the human race. Now as to the method after the master prover deals out these vials, each prover takes a single dose of the medicine and waits to see if the single dose takes effect. If he is sensitive to that medicine a single dose will produce symptoms, and then those symptoms must not be interfered with; they should be allowed to go their own way. In the proving of an acute remedy, like *Aconitum napellus*; the instructor, who knows something about the effect of the medicine, may be able to say to the class: "If you are going to get effects from this remedy you will get those effects in the next three to four days." It will not be necessary to wait longer than that for *Aconitum napellus, Nux vomica,* or *Ignatia amara,* but longer for *Sulphur* or some of the antipsorics. If we were attempting to prove a remedy like Silicate of Alumina, the master-prover would advise the class not to interfere with the medicine for at least thirty days, because its prodrome may be thirty days.

It is highly important to wait until the possible prodrome of a given remedy is surely passed. If it is a short-acting remedy, the action will come speedily. We must bear in mind the prodrome, the period of progress and the period of decline when studying the Materia Medica as well as when studying miasms. The master-prover will usually be able to indicate to the class whether they should wait a short time or a long time before taking another dose, and from this the class will only know whether the drug to be proved is acute or chronic.

If the first dose of medicine produces no effect, and enough time has been allowed to be sure that the prover is not sensitive to it, the next best thing to do is to create a sensitiveness to it. If we examine into the effects of poisons, we find those who have once been poisoned by Rhus are a dozen times more sensitive than before. Those who have been poisoned by Arsenic are extremely sensitive to Arsenic after they allow the first effects to pass off. If they continue, however, to keep on with the first effects they become less sensitive to it, so that they require larger and larger doses to take effect. This is a rule with all poisonous substances that are capable of affecting the human system markedly. Now, when the time has passed by which the prover knows he is not sensitive to that remedy, that he has not received an action from the dose (and perhaps in the class of forty you will not get more than one or two that will make a proving from the 30th potency) to make the proving and to intensify the effect, dissolve the medicine in water and have him take every two hours for 24 to 48 hours, unless symptoms arise sooner. By this means the prodromal period is shortened. The medicine seems to be intensified by the repetition, and the patient is brought under the influence, dynamically, of that remedy. As soon as the symptoms begin to show, it is time to cease taking the remedy.

No danger comes from giving the remedy in this way; danger comes from taking it for a few days and then stopping it, and then taking it again. For instance, say you are proving *Arsenicum album*; you find that you are not all sensitive to it, and after waiting thirty days you start out again and take it in water, for three to four days, and the symptoms arise; now wait. So long as you discontinue it, it will not do any damage. Now, the symptoms begin to arise; wait, and let the image-producing effect of *Arsenicum album* wear off; let it come and spread and go away of itself; do not interfere with it; if you do interfere with it, the interference should be only by a true antidote; you should never interfere with it by a repetition of dose. That is one of the most dangerous things. If the *Arsenicum album* symptoms are coming and showing clearly, and at the end of a week or ten days you say: "Let us brighten this up a little, and do this thing more thoroughly," and to accomplish this you take a great deal more, you will engraft upon your constitution in that way the Arsenicum diathesis, from which you will never be cured. You are breaking right into the cycles of that remedy and it is a dangerous thing to do. At times that has been done and the provers have carried the effects of their proving to the end of their days. If you leave this Arsenical state alone it will pass off entirely, and the prover is very often left much better for it. A proving properly conducted will improve the health of anybody; it will help to turn things into order. It was Hahnemanns advice to young men to make provings.

Another portion of the class will not get symptoms, no matter how they abuse the remedy, and if it be *Arsenicum* they will have to take a crude dose of it to get any effect, and then the symptoms given forth are only the toxic effects, from which little can be gained. The toxicological results of poisons are provings of the grossest character: they do not give the finer details. For instance, you give *Opium* in such large doses that it immediately poisons; you see nothing but the grosser, overwhelming symptoms; the irregular, stertorous breathing, the unconsciousness, the contracted pupil and the mottled face and the irregular heart. The details are not there, you only have a view of the most common things.

The reproving of remedies is of great value. The Vienna Society did not fully endorse Hahnemann's provings. This society thought it impossible that such wonderful things could be brought out upon the sensations of people. The society did not endorse the 30th potency that was recommended by Hahnemann for proving. So this society gathered itself together and resolved to prove remedies, and to test the 30th potency, and it so happened that the society was honest. *Natrium muriaticum, Thuja occidentalis* and other remedies were proved, and W-was honest enough to say that although his convictions were decidedly against the provings he had to admit that the symptoms gathered from the 30th potency were very strong. The Vienna Society demonstrated by these reprovings that the polychrests of Hahnemann had been fully proved. Their provings of the 30th of *Natrium muriaticum* was a wonderful revelation of them; but W-, in spite of this result, held on to his prejudices. He acknowledged that he was wrong; but he continued to use potencies lower than the 15th. He could not get his mind elevated to the 30th; his prejudice was too strong. Dunham says of some of these, that in spite of the fact that they had seen better results from the 30th and higher potencies even, they were so prejudiced they could not bring themselves to a state of yielding. As Dunham humorously expressed it, "they are ossified in their cerebral convolutions as well as in their bony structure." That is to say, their minds were inelastic, they could not expand. We talk from appearance when we say the eyes are closed;

it is the mind that is closed, the understanding that is closed.

Read § 107-112.—When the patient is under the poisonous influence of a drug it does not seem to flow in the direction of his life action, but when reaction comes then the lingering effects of the drug seems to flow, as it were, in the stream of the vital action. Then the symptoms that arise are of the best order, and hence it is necessary in proving a drug to take such a portion of the drug only as will disturb and not suspend, as it will flow in the stream of the vital order, in the order of the economy, establishing slightly perverted action, and causing symptoms, without suspending action, as we would, for example, with a large dose of Opium. When a state of suspension exists in the dynamic economy, then we have a beclouding of all the activities of the economy; so giving a large dose of medicine to palliate pains and sufferings is dangerous. We have a suspension of the vital order when we give a medicine that does not flow in the stream of the vital influx, homoeopathy looks towards the administration of medicines that are given for the purpose of either creating order, and then always in the higher potencies, or for the purpose of disturbing, and then in the lower potencies. We should never resort to crude drugs for provings, unless for a momentary or temporary experiment. It should not be followed up, and no great weight should be put upon the provings that are made from the crude medicines. They only at best give a fragmentary idea. Unless the proving that has been made with strong doses becomes enlarged with the symptoms from small doses the information remains fragmentary and useless. If we had only the poisonous effects of *Opium*, we would be able only to use it in those conditions that simulate the poisonous effects of *Opium*, like apoplexy.

There are some prescribers who teach that for the primary effect one potency must be used and for the secondary effect another must be used. No such distinction need be made. I have many times been at the bedside of apoplectic patients when death would have followed had not the homoeopathic remedy been administered. I have been at the bedside of some when the pulse was flickering, when the eye was glazed, when the countenance was besotted, stertorous breathing coming on, frothing at the mouth, and in a few minutes after the administration of Opium c.m. I have seen the patient go into a sound sleep, remain quiet and rest, wake up to consciousness, and go on to recovery. *Alumina* has a similar state of stupor resembling apoplexy, and hence it is that *Alumina* and *Opium* are antidotes to each other. I remember a case of apoplexy once that puzzled many physicians for some days, and I was puzzled, too. The patient was in a profound stupor. *Opium* was administered by the physician in charge before I arrived, and it stopped the stertorous breathing, but the patient remained unconscious. Finally it was observed that one side was moving, whilst the other side had not moved for many days, and that on the paralyzed side there was fever, while on the well side there was no fever. That was observed after careful examination for many days. I asked the doctor if he did not consider that the natural state of a paralyzed side would be coldness; he thought so too. The whole paralyzed side of this patient had a feverish feeling to the hand, the other side was normal. That seemed to be the only strange thing in the case; no speech, no effort to do anything, no action of the bowels; a do nothing case. Upon a careful study of the Materia Medica, I came to the conclusion that *Alumina* was suited to the case, and in twelve hours after taking a dose of *Alumina* in a high potency that fever subsided on the paralyzed side and the patient returned to consciousness.

Classroom Notes

Study of Provings

The best way to study a remedy is to make a proving of it. The guidelines to provings are as follows:
1.   Before entering into a proving, the class of provers should spend a week in writing down all the symptoms that the prover supposes he is victim of. This is the *baseline record*.
2.   A *master prover* is decided upon, who will prepare for the

proving a substance unknown to the class and all the provers.

3. He will *prepare the drug* from mother tincture to 30th potency putting a portion of that potency into a separate vial for each member of the class.

4. *Provers do not know* what they are taking and they are requested not to *make known to each other* their symptoms.

5. Each prover takes a single dose of the medicine and waits to see if the *single dose takes effect*. Wait for 3-4 days to a maximum of 30 days.

6. If the first dose of the medicine produces no effect, dissolve the medicine in water and have him take every two hours for 24 to 48 hours, unless symptoms arise.

7. As soon as the *symptoms begin to show* either after first dose or repeated doses. Its time to *stop taking the remedy*.

8. To brighten up the effects if you take more of the medicine you will engraft upon the constitution a *great deal of medicinal diathesis* of which you may never be cured.

9. During the proving use of any other *strong medicine is prohibited*.

10. **Interpretation:**

    (a) Closely *watch the order* of appearance of symptoms.

    (b) When the *original symptoms are modified*, note whether they are cured or exaggerated. If symptoms are not changed by the medicine delete them from the proving.

    (c) If a remedy takes a marked hold of a prover, all the chronic symptoms will subside, but when a proving only takes a partial hold it may cure only a few symptoms.

    (d) These *few symptoms* added to the *symptoms* that the *other provers have felt*, will go to makeup the *chronic effects of the remedy*, which may be said to be said to be the effect of the remedy upon the human race.

LECTURE XXIX

§ 117. Idiosyncrasies

THE study of the *idiosyncrasies* is closely related to homoeopathy. The usual explanation of the term is, an over sensitiveness to one thing or a few things. It does not apply to the general susceptibility in feeble constitutions where patients are susceptible to all things, over-susceptible and over impressed by simple annoyances. In the old school idiosyncrasies relate to certain patients who are known in every practitioner's practice as oversensitive. One oversensitive cannot take Opium for his pains, because of the congestion it produces, because of dangerous symptoms; he is oversensitive to it and has complication from a very small dose even and the physician is compelled not to administer it. Another patient cannot tolerate Quinine in chills and fever; the primary action of Quinine makes him alarmingly sick; where another individual may take 15 grains. One who has an idiosyncrasy to Quinine cannot take one-quarter of a grain without having an over-action of that drug -a state of quininism. The homoeopath recognizes of wide range in susceptibility, including things that the allopath is not acquainted with. There may be a chronic idiosyncrasy from a chronic miasm and an acute idiosyncrasy from an acute miasm. There are certain individuals in every community that cannot ride in the country because of their susceptibility to hay fever; others cannot bear the smell of flowers in the room because of becoming sick; some will get sick from the smell of roses. I have known a number of patients who became sick in this way. It is common enough, and the sickness is known by the name of rose cold or rose fever. I have a patient who cannot have dry lavender flowers in the house without coming down with coryza. She is disturbed by two or three things in this way, and will go looking about to see which one of those things is in the house. I had another patient who could not have peaches in the room without becoming sick; one of the symptoms that he had was diarrhoea. This over sensibility is very important and it explains in a measure the susceptibility to the remedy that will cure. If an idiosyncrasy to the remedy is not present, the patient will not be susceptible enough to be cured. The state in which he becomes sensitive enough to a drug to cure him is very analogous to these idiosyncrasies above mentioned. Think what susceptibility man must have to the remedy that cures him, when, it cures in the very high attenuations that we use.

There are acquired idiosyncrasies and idiosyncrasies that are born with a patient. Those that are congenital and those that come from poisons are most difficult. In *Rhus toxicodendron* poisoning those that have once been affected by handling it are so sensitive to it that if they go within a quarter of a mile of the vine, though they cannot detect it with the nose, yet in a few days they will come down with a case of *Rhus toxicodendron* poisoning. A very high potency of *Rhus toxicodendron* will sometimes remove that susceptibility and a dose of *Rhus toxicodendron* c.m. or m.m. will often check the acute poisoning from *Rhus toxicodendron*: but if you find that the patient has been born with a sensitivity to *Rhus toxicodendron*, while *Rhus toxicodendron* may palliate a few times it will finally cease to help him. When one is born with this sensitivity it is very tenacious and will sometimes persist, in spite of our best endeavors, to the end of life. If eradicated at all, it requires an antipsoric to get to the bottom of it. Hay fever is brought on in the fall and is supposed to be caused by the patient's over-sensitiveness to irritants that develop about that time; sometimes it is attributed to the hay that is curing in the fields at that time, sometimes to the different weeds that grow up then. Such patients have often been able to ferret out the thing that they are susceptible to. But psora is at the bottom of all these troubles. Patients getting up from typhoid fever have often idiosyncrasies, and the chronic miasms are responsible for these, just as psora is prior to the sore eyes from scarlet fever. Sequelae are miasmatic, they are simply the outcroppings of chronic miasms.

There are persons who are sensitive, not merely to one or a few things, but to all things; oversensitive to the high potencies, oversensitive in taste, oversensitive to light, and a great many other things. This is a constitutional state; the patient is born with it. There are persons in whom you will see the sensitiveness only when you go away from the plane of nutrition into the plane of dynamics. You will see for instance patients who will sit at the table and crave common salt; want lots of salt upon their food, and never seem able to get just exactly what they need. They eat plenty of common salt and remain sick, growing thinner all the time. This is on the nutritive plane; the crude common salt is taken with the food. Now you administer the c.m. to such a patient, and it makes that patient sick, producing a violent aggravation.

This is where a food sustains a curative relation upon a higher plane. We step out of the nutritive plane into the plane of dynamics, the plane of disease-cause and cure.

Take *Calcarea carbonica* as an instance. We see the allopath and crude medicine man give to certain babies, that are slow in forming bone and teeth and have open fontanelles, lime water in milk, and the more lime water he gives them the less bone they make. Here is a bone-salt inanition, a non-assimilation of lime. A dose of *Calcarea carbonica* very high will enable that child to take all the lime that it needs from the food that it eats. The remedy given on the dynamic plane cause a digestion and assimilation of the lime naturally present in the food. You may feed lime in crude form, and no benefit ever come; the child goes on withering and emaciating.

In such non-assimilating patients the symptoms of *Calcarea carbonica* or *Natrium muriaticum* appear, calling the attention of the intelligent physician to the fact that the child needs *Calcarea carbonica* or *Natrium muriaticum*. We know very well that we do not build bone with the c.m. potency of lime, it simply corrects internal disorder and causes the outward forms of the body to flow into order. The turning into order of the internal establishes the nutritive principle from the internal to the external. So that we can see the wider ranges that idiosyncrasy or susceptibility has in homoeopathy.

Here we might undertake to coin a word, viz. : - homoeopathicity; what does it mean? Homoeopathicity is the relation between the homoeopathic remedy and the patient who has been cured. When the homoeopathic remedy has acted properly, when it has cured the patient, it has demonstrated that it was homoeopathically related to the case; so that the relation, when it was sustained, may be called the homoeopathicity, and it is demonstrated by administering the remedy. It is true that we can have what would be called a normal homoeopathicity, a normal state, and that state exaggerated. That state exaggerated is where the patient is over-sensitive to the curative remedy, and it not only establishes a curative relation, but before curing produces an exaggeration of the symptoms of the patient. A remedy demonstrates its similitude to a case by curing. Homoeopathic physicians use the word simillimum. The simillimum might be called that remedy that has cured the patient, but in advance of curing that case it is only what *appears* to be the most similar; a medicine cannot be called the simillimum until it has cured.

It is worthy of consideration to discover the difference between a poison taken upon the nutritive plane, that is, in crude substance, and a poison taken upon the dynamic plane. A poison upon the nutritive plane is usually not very deep, is more superficial, it relates more to external things, to the body and tissues, while the poison taken upon the dynamic plane may last a lifetime. The miasms are of such a character. Poison taken upon the nutritive plane may bring about a life-long effect upon an individual, owing to susceptibility. The small doses of *Arsenicum album* will establish an *Arsenicum album* poisoning that will last a lifetime, but this is nowhere so deep as will be represented by the higher potencies of *Arsenicum album*. To poison a patient with the higher potencies there is generally required something of susceptibility, while to poison patients upon the nutritive plane susceptibility is not required; any patient can be brought under the influence of a poison given upon the nutritive plane.

Here is another difference. Substances that are inert and substances that we can use as food on the nutritive plane may become poisonous upon the dynamic plane to those that are susceptible. So that there is no substance that may not be a poison in the higher and highest potencies. This gives us a distinction between crude and dynamic poisons that you will do well to think about.

Now from all this we are led to see that if there were no state of susceptibility, no such condition as idiosyncrasy, there could be no homoeopathy. If there were no susceptibility, there would be no sickness and no need of homoeopathy.

Susceptibility underlies all contagion and all cure. So that cause and cure, the cause of sickness and the cure of sickness, knock at the same door. They flow in the same way because of the immaterial or simple substance. All disease is in primitive substance, or first substance; all cure of disease must also be in simple substance. In olden times we used to think that all substances capable of extinguishing the vital force, or which overcome the vital force, were poisons; that in itself is a crude idea of a poison. Any substance capable of impressing itself upon the economy of man sufficiently to cause death, or to create a disorder in the economy, may be called a poison. The definition will apply to both dynamic and crude poisons. Poison presents two problems: an external problem and an internal problem. The external deals with the question of quantity, the internal with the question of quality. A dynamis cannot be considered from the standpoint of weights and measures, but from quality. Crude substances are considered from the standpoint of quantity, from weights and measures.

This is only a beginning to set you thinking. This subject leads into the study of protection as well. There are two forms of protection from sickness. Man is protected from sickness in two ways, by homoeopathy and by use. The physician and the nurse who go into the district of yellow fever or typhoid or diphtheria or smallpox, who keep busy, who have, in the highest sense of the word, the true love of the use, who have gone into the work as mediums of mercy, will be largely protected just simply from their love of the work, from their delight in it. They have no fear. Fear is an overwhelming cause of sickness; those who fall prey to fear are likely to become sick, but those who face disease with no fear are likely to remain well; they do sometimes fall sick, it is true, but I believe it is because they begin to have fear in the work.

The other and greater prophylactic is the homoeopathic remedy. After working in an epidemic for a few weeks, you will find perhaps that half-a-dozen remedies are daily indicated and one of these in a large number of cases than any other. This one remedy seems to be the best suited to the general nature of the sickness. Now you will find that for prophylaxis there is required a less degree of similitude than is necessary for curing. A remedy will not have to be so similar to prevent disease as to cure it, and these remedies in daily use will enable you to prevent a large number of people from becoming sick. We must look to homoeopathy for our protection as well as for our cure.

Classroom Notes

Idiosyncrasies

1. *Idiosyncrasies* are defined as over-sensitiveness to one or few things.
2. There are *acquired* and *congenital* idiosyncrasies.
3. Congenital idiosyncrasies are hard to eradicate but if ever they are, it is only by anti-Psorics.
4. The over-sensitivity is very important and it explains a measure of susceptibility (to the remedy that shall cure).

5.   If the Idiosyncrasy to the remedy is not present, the patient
      will not be susceptible enough to be cured.

Poisons

1.   Any substance capable of impressing itself upon the inter-
      nal state of man sufficiently to cause death, or to create a
      disorder in the internal state, may be called a poison.

2.   This definition will apply to both dynamic and crude
      poisons.

3.   A poison upon the nutritive plane is usually not very deep
      i.e. it relates to most external things, to the body and tissues.
      Short term effects of poisons, on nutritive plane are not
      dependent on susceptibility. Poisons taken upon the nutri-
      tive plane may bring about a life long effect upon an indi-
      vidual owing to susceptibility.

4.   A poison taken upon the dynamic plane may last a lifetime.
      To effect a patient with higher potencies generally requires
      susceptibility.

5.   Substances that are inert (*Lycopodium* for instance) and
      substances that we can use as food (*Asafoetida*) on the
      nutritive plane may become poisonous upon the dynamic
      plane to those who are susceptible.

LECTURE XXX

§ 118, ETC. Individualization

COMPARISON, individualization, and difference in the nature of things most similar, are points that must be carefully considered. The substitution of one remedy for another cannot be thought of, or entertained in homoeopathy. The homoeopathic physician must individualize, he must discriminate. He must individualize things widely dissimilar in one way, yet similar in other ways. Take for instance the two remedies, *Secale cornutum* and *Arsenicum album*; they are both chilly, but the patient wants all the covers off and wants the cold air in *Secale cornutum*, and he wants all things hot in *Arsenicum album*. The two remedies thus separate at once; they are wholly dissimilar as to the general state, whilst wholly similar as to particulars. A mere book-worm symptom hunter would see no difference between *Secale cornutum* and *Arsenicum album*. You go to the bedside of a case of peritonitis, and you will find the abdomen distended, the patient restless; you will find him often vomiting blood and passing blood from the anus; you will find horrible burning with the distended abdomen, unquenchable thirst, dry, red tongue, lightning-like pulse. Well, *Arsenicum album* and *Secale cornutum* have all these things equally; they both have these things in high degree; but when *Secale cornutum* is indicated he wants all the covers off, wants to be cold, wants cold applications, wants the windows open; cannot tolerate the heat, and the warm room makes him worse. If *Arsenicum album* is indicated in such a case, he wants to be wrapped up warmly, even in the month of July, wants hot food and hot drinks. The whole Materia Medica is full of these things and is based upon this kind of individualization.

Without the generals of a case no man can practice homoeopathy, for without these no man can individualize and see distinctions. After gathering all the particulars, one strong general rules out one remedy and rules in another. Physicians by the questions they ask often show that they have not been able to grasp this idea of individualization. They pick out two symptoms, or one symptom common to two remedies, and say, "Now, both of these remedies have this same symptom, how are you going to tell them apart?" Well, if you are acquainted with the Materia Medica, with the art of individualization, you will at once easily see how to get the generals; the generals of one are so and so, and the generals of the other are so and so, and this will enable you to distinguish one of these remedies as best adapted to the constitution, when the two remedies have the one symptom in any equal degree. Now, this rules out the idea of substitution. If one does not work, they say, try all down the list alphabetically, until you hit it. Why a remedy that has never been known to produce that symptom may cure the case, because it is more similar to the *generals* of that case than any other. This is the art of applying the Materia Medica. Many times a patient brings out that which is so strange and rare that it has never been found in any remedy. You have to examine the whole case and see which remedy of all remedies is most similar to the patient himself. From beginning to end, the homoeopath must study the patient. If he become conversant with symptoms apart from the patient, he will not be successful.

Par. 118 reads: "Each medicine produces particular effects in the body of man, and no other medicinal substance can create any that are precisely similar." That is the beginning of a doctrine showing that there can be no substitution. There are cases that are so mixed that man, no matter how much he studies, cannot see the distinctions; but, remember one thing, there is one remedy that is needed in the case, whether it is known or not; it is needed in the case, and it has no substitute, for that remedy differs from all other medicines, just as this individual differs from all other individuals. It may be that we cannot see that it is needed, it may not appear to be indicated, but it is needed all the same, though the intimation may not have come to the eye or ear of the physician. That shows the necessity of waiting and watching. In homoeopathy medicines can never replace each other, nor one be as good as another.

As we hasten along with this subject, we find in Par. 122 Hahnemann says: "In circumstances of this nature on which depend the certitude of the medical art, and the welfare of future generations, it is necessary to employ only medicines that are well-known." Purity is important, medicines as they are proved should be kept unmodified and preserved and possessed of their full energy. Now, it is important that you shall use the same substances, as nearly as possible, as were proved. Among the potencies that we are using here as high potencies, made by Fincke and others, we have in a large number of instances the very identical substances that were proved by the provers. It is important not to change. A plant bearing the same name as the one proved, but grown in a different climate and on a different soil, should not be used. Procure the one that was proved originally. Fincke recognized this when he procured the substances that Hering proved. We have the same *Lachesis mutus* that Hering proved. I have a sample of the original *Lachesis mutus* that I am preserving in a little vial marked with Hering's own name. The medicine should be well-known; its history should be well-known, with all the steps and details. The question of potentization should be taken into account, the different hands they have been through; all the little particulars of our high potencies should be well known. You should not be careless in this and not gather potencies from Tom, Dick and Harry. When able, go to headquarters and get your potencies.

Hahnemann writes in Par. 144: "A Materia Medica of this nature shall be free from all conjecture, fiction or gratuitous assertion it shall contain nothing but the pure language of nature, the results of a careful and faithful research." We have formed, built and established the Materia Medica by provings upon the healthy, and observations that are pure and honestly made. Par. 145: "We ought certainly to be acquainted with the pure action of a vast number of medicines upon the healthy body, to be able to find homoeopathy remedies against each of the innumerable forms of disease that besiege mankind; that is to say, to find out artificial morbific powers that resemble them." At the present time it will rarely be found that a fully developed disease has not its simillimum, its remedy and cure, in our Materia Medica. It is only those mixed cases that are not developed that puzzle us.

Classroom Notes

Individualisation

1.   Comparison, Individualisation, and Differentiation in nature of things most similar are those points that must be carefully considered.

2.   A Homeopathic physician must individualise.

3.   To individualise he must discriminate.

4.   Without generals no man can individualise.

5.   One strong general can rule out one remedy and include one in.

6.   If the generals match and particular don't, give the remedy that matches the generals.

7.   In the mixed cases, where discrimination and individualisation is not possible, one must wait and watch.

8.   Use medicines that are well known.

9.   Use the plant for the same area where remedy was proved.

10.   Individualisation is the art of applying the Materia Medica.

§ 146: "The third point in the duty of the physician is to employ those medicines whose pure effects have been proved upon a healthy person in the manner best suited to the cure of natural diseases homoeopathically." We will take this up in our next talk.

This third point in the duty of the physician referred to in § 146 really takes up the balance of the *Organon*.

§ 147: Of all these medicines that one whose symptoms bear the greatest resemblance to the totality of those which characterize any particular natural disease ought to be the most appropriate and certain homoeopathic remedy that can be employed; it is the specific remedy in this case of disease." It is not an uncommon thing in this advanced day of science to read of specific remedies. The old school distinctly affirms that there are only three or four specifics, but almost every off-shoot who starts at something for himself has to a great extent the idea of specifics in him. One of the first things the quack physician seems inclined to do is to commence advertising specifics for headache, for diarrhœa, for this or that. This is altoghether opposed to homoeopathy. There are no specifics in homoeopathy except at the bedside of a patient when the remedy has been wrought out with great endeavor and care. Then it may be said that medicine, which is found to be similar to the symptoms, which characterize this disease, is specific.

Now, please note that there is an emphatic sense in that word "characterizes." It is no ordinary expression. We have read in the earlier portions of the *Organon* that the disease makes itself known to the physician by signs and symptoms, and that the totality of the symptoms is the sole representation of the disease, to the physician; but that totality has to be studies to ascertain what there is, among all the symptoms, that *characterizes* the disease, or marks the symptoms as peculiar.

Now Hahnemann commences to analyze the totality of the symptoms for the purpose of giving it character. It has been said in these lectures that it is necessary to do that, that the information that leads up to characterizing is really the information that makes the homoeopathic physician wise, by which he has the ability to intelligently understand that which he has to treat. That medicine, which is best, adapted is the most similar, but you cannot demonstrate beforehand that is the specific homoeopathic remedy; for you may be deceived in your idea of the nature of the case. But when that remedy has acted, then it may be seen that remedy was homoeopathic, or specific, or that it was not homoeopathic. You have no idea as to what remedy will be homoeopathic to the case until you have examined all the symptoms, and then proceed to find out that which characterizes.

Put that word *characterizes* in large type, in red letters. You can not dwell sufficiently long upon that, because it grows greater and grander with every study of the case, that idea of the characteristic. What is there in this case which makes it an individual, what is there in it that makes it unlike any that ever existed? In the case of the remedy ascertain that which characterizes it. When these two occur before the perception, before man's mind, so that he can think upon them, and he realizes that the remedy is the most similar of all in the Materia Medica, then he is assured that that remedy will cure, and it only requires to be administered to prove that it is the specific. The homoeopathicity is thus sustained, the similitude has been borne out by the medicine having cured. We cannot have the demonstration that the remedy is homoeopathic until it cures the sick man; we may only presume that it is homoeopathic, or say it appears to us that it is homoeopathic, because that which is characteristic of the disease is most similar of all other things to that which is characteristic of that remedy, or vice versa. We may reasonably assume that that remedy is the specific, but the homoeopathicity can only be demonstrated by cure. So it does not make a remedy homoeopathic simply to be carried in my case. Homoeopathic remedies are not homoeopathic simply because they have been used by a homoeopath. Remedies are not homoeopathic because potentized and attenuated or prepared after the fashion of our school.

What constitutes a remedy homoeopathic? The answer is: It has demonstrated its curative relation to the patient, after having been prescribed in accordance with his symptoms, the recovery taking place in the proper direction, from above downward, from within out, and in the reverse order of the symptoms. That constitutes a remedy homoeopathic, and that constitutes the prescription homoeopathic. It is then a specific remedy, and in no other sense can a remedy be called a specific. Hahnemann gives his theory of cure in paragraph 148, but you are not compelled to adopt it. Hahnemann himself says it is only a theory, and he offers it as simply the best in view, but not as binding upon you to accept.

But Paragraph 149 is something that must be accepted, that is, it must be known and then accepted because it is true. It is a general statement of the results of the homoeopathic remedy in the cure of disease. The rejection of this paragraph must effect a separation amongst those who do not believe, and those who do believe. "When a proper application of the homoeopathic remedy has been made, the acute disease which is to be cured, however malignant and painful it may be, subsides in a few hours, if recent, and in a few days, if it is somewhat older," etc.

From this I am placed under the plain necessity of acknowledging that if under my treatment such diseases do not subside. I have not found the right remedy. That will force the honest homoeopathic physician to seek the proper remedy. Let not the blame be placed upon the failure of the system and of law and order, but let it be placed upon the one who practices it. Just so sure as you find the homoeopathic remedy in a case of scarlet fever, just so sure you will see that fever fall and that child improve; while the rash will remain out, nothing of the malignancy of the case will remain, in an ordinary case of scarlet fever; we find that in a few days the child is so much better he wants to go to school. But then we treat the child and not the fever. Just so sure as the physician has in mind the rash of scarlet fever or of measles as the main element of the disease, he will make a failure, and the patient will not recover so speedily; but as a matter of fact, the homoeopathic physician prescribes for the patient on that which characterizes the sickness, even though it be what is called a self-limiting disease.

§ 150. This treats of one of the difficulties we have to contend with. "If a patient complains of slightly accessory symptoms which have just appeared, the physician ought not to take this state of things for a perfect malady that seriously demands medicinal aid, etc., etc. It is right for you, when your patients are under constitutional treatment, to prescribe for a cold, but only when it is not an ordinary one. If the cold is likely to cause serious trouble, then you must prescribe for it; slight indisposition, however, should not receive remedies. You will have patients that will come to you at every change of the wind, at every attack of snuffles the baby has at every little headache or every little pain. If you then proceed to change your remedy or prescribe for each one of these little spells of indisposition, you will, in the course of a little while, have such a state of disorder in the individual that you will wonder what is the matter with this patient. You had better give her no medicine at all, and if she is wise and strong and can feel confidence you can say to her that she does not need medicine for this attack; but occasionally give her a dose of constitutional medicine when these little attacks are not on. While you are young and cannot hold these patients with an iron grasp, when they come to you, you had better give them placebo, and let the indisposition pass off of itself. Watch it, however, and it may at the close develop some constitutional manifestation and throw light upon the patient that you have been treating. On the other hand, it is an easy patient that you have been treating. On the other hand, it is an easy matter to prescribe for severe acute diseases; they are decisive, they strongly manifest their symptoms, they are sharp cut in their expressions, the symptoms are prominent, and you will not be confused as you will be in the slight indispositions. The slight indispositions are nondescript; you do not know what to do for them. In vain you seek to find that which characterizes them, and hence it is doubtful about any remedy, that is administered being of any value. You will be astonished after prescribing a number of years, and your patients have gained confidence in you, that when they come in with these little trivial ailments they won't have them after a few powders of sugar. They will say : "Doctor, my trouble went off splendidly." This is what is meant by letting the little things alone. Severe diseases exhibit a strong degree of symptoms, and hence you have something to do. Paragraph 151. "But if the few symptoms of which the patient complains are very violent, the physician who attentively observed him will generally discover many others which are less developed and which furnish a perfect picture of the malady."

Classroom Notes

Characteristics

[Para: 147]

1. By the idea of characteristic we mean; what is there in this case, which makes it an individual and what is there in it that makes it unlike any other case that ever existed.
2. That which is characteristic symptom of the disease must be similar of all other things to that which is characteristic symptom of that remedy.
3. All other symptoms (properly selected) must be used to discriminate between similar remedy (diffrential diagnosis of remedies).

[Para: 148]
Hahnemann gives his theory of cure and you are not compelled
to adopt it.

[Para: 149]
Accept what is said here. If a proper application of Homeopathic
medicine is done in an acute disease then the acute disease that is
to be cured, however painful, it subsides in few hours if recent
and in a few days if it is somewhat older.

[Para: 150]
What to do in chronic diseases when *accessory symptoms* appear
after a medicine is prescribed?
1. If the symptoms are likely to cause serious trouble then
    prescribe for them.
2. Do not prescribe for slight indisposition or give *placebo*
    and let the indisposition pass by itself.
3. Watch these symptoms closely as in the end they may
    develop some constitutional manifestations and throw light
    upon the patient being treated.

LECTURE XXXII

The Value of Symptoms

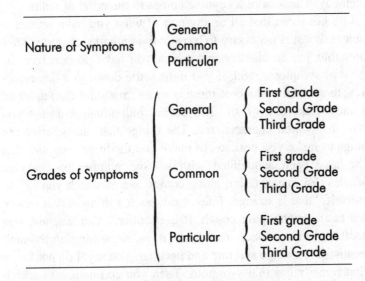

Nature of Symptoms		General
		Common
		Particular

Grades of Symptoms	General	First Grade
		Second Grade
		Third Grade
	Common	First grade
		Second Grade
		Third Grade
	Particular	First grade
		Second Grade
		Third Grade

§ 153 IS the one that teaches more particularly how the process of individualization or discrimination shall be carried out. It treats of characteristics, it treats of grades. The homoeopathic physician may think he has his case written out very well, but he does not know whether he has or not until he has mastered the idea of this paragraph. He may have page after page of symptoms, and not know what the remedy is, and if he takes the record to master the master will say: "You have no case!" "Why, I have plenty of symptoms." "But you have no case. You have left your case out; you have left the image of the sickness out, because you have failed to get anything that characterizes it. You have plenty of symptoms, but have not anything characteristic. You have not taken your case properly." Now, after you have mastered this paragraph you will know whether you have taken your case properly, you will know whether you have something to present to a master, a likeness of something. The lack of this knowledge is the cause of non-success with the majority homoeopathic physicians. There are a great many homoeopathic physicians that prescribe and tinker a long time with their cases, and will ask you what a characteristic is, and if it is some one peculiar thing that guides to a remedy. The idea of a keynote comes to the mind of many.

I do not mean that all or any part of what you have written is useless, but it is necessary to have individualizing characteristics to enable you to classify that which you have, to perceive the value of symptoms, and, if you must settle down to a few remedies, to ascertain which of these is more important than another, or most important of all. You cannot individualize unless you have that which characterizes. The things that characterize are things to make you hesitate, to make you meditate. Suppose that you have been acquainted with a large number of cases of measles, for instance, but along comes one of which you say to yourself, "that is strange: I never saw such a thing as that before in a case of whooping cough. It is peculiar." You hesitate, you meditate, and at once recognize it as something individual, because it is strange and rare and peculiar. You say, I do not know what remedy has that symptom. Then you commence to search your repertory, or consult those of more experience, and you find in the repertory, or upon consultation, that such a medicine has that thing as a strong feature, as a high grade symptom, and it is as peculiar in the remedy as in your patient, though you have never seen it before. You may have seen a hundred cases of measles without seeing that very thing. That peculiar thing that you see in measles relates to the patient and not to the disease; and as the sole duty of the physician is to heal the sick that peculiar thing will open the whole case to the remedy. When you find that the remedy has than symptoms along with the other symptoms, you must attach some importance to it, and when there are two or three of these peculiar symptoms they form the *characteristic features.*

What would you think would constitute a *common* symptom? We shall at once see that the common symptoms are those that appear in all cases of measles, that you would expect to find in measles. It would be strange to have measles without any rash; that would be peculiar. We know that the absence of rash is a striking state of affairs and means trouble, and is peculiar. Either it is not measles, or the absence of the rash is a serious state. Suppose it is a fever. The patient has intense heat an ordinary fever coming in the afternoon and running through the night, with hot hands and feet, high temperature, dry tongue. etc. What would you say concerning the presence of absence of thirst? You would say it is *common* if he has thirst, because almost anybody who has fever would want water. Nothing is so natural to put fire out with as water, and the absence of thirst in a fever is strange, is rare and uncommon, peculiar and striking. You will ask yourself at once is it not strange that he does not have thirst with such a high temperature? You at once strike to the remedies that are thirstless. You would not think of hunting up a remedy that has thirst.

So the absence of the striking features of disease constitutes a peculiarity that relates to the patient. Well, then, that which is pathognomonic is common, because it is common in that disease, but an absence of the pathognomonic characterizes that particular disease in that patient, and therefore means the patient, and in proportion as you have that class of symptoms just in that proportion you have things that characterize the patient, and the specific remedy for the patient will be the simillimum. It is necessary to know sickness, not from pathology, not from physical diagnosis, no matter how important these branches are, but by symptoms, the language of nature.

A true homoeopathic prescription cannot be made on pathology or morbid anatomy; because provings have never been pushed in that direction. Pathology gives us the results of disease, and not the language of nature appealing to the intelligent physician. Symptomatolgy is the true subject to know. No man, who is only conversant with morbid anatomy and pathognomonic symptoms, can make homoeopathic prescriptions. In addition to diagnostic ability he must have a peculiar knowledge; that is, he must be acquainted with the manner of expression of each and every disease. He must know just how each disease expresses itself in language and appearance and sensations. He must know just how every remedy affects mankind in the memory and understanding and will, because there are no other things that the remedy can act upon as to the mind, and he must know how the remedy affects functions, because there are no other ways in which the remedy affects the body of man. Now, if he knows how diseases express themselves in signs and symptoms, then he knows what constitutes an individual disease a little different from all others. It is the peculiar way that the same disease affects different patients that makes the symptoms strange, peculiar and rare. That which is pathognomonic in the remedy is that which you will study out most, because it is that which is related to the patient. Such is the state of mind that the homoeopathic physicians must keep themselves in, in order to begin this study, and when they have begun to think in this way they can then study the symptoms of the disease as to grade.

The symptoms of the remedies must be studied especially with respect to *order on grade*. To look upon them as all alike, because they appear to be all on the same level, is to be unable to make distinctions. One symptom with some physicians is as good as another. It is a fact that symptoms, to a great extent, are upon a sliding scale. What is peculiar in one remedy is not in any degree peculiar in another. While it may be peculiar in a chronic case to have thirst, it is not so in a fever. That which is true in many respects in a chronic miasms may be the very opposite in an acute case. The chronic miasms are the very opposite in their character and order to the acute miasms, and this is a fact that the homoeopathic physician must know.

If you had a striking case of inflammation of the parotid gland, the patient says : "Do not press upon it, because it is very sore," how would you classify that, as common or strange? If you think but a moment, you will see that it would be a very strange thing of a highly inflamed gland not to be sore, and that soreness upon pressure is not something to be prescribed for, but something to be known, to be taken into the general view of the case, and the remedy indicated in the case would be suitable if it have inflammation and soreness of the gland; there is nothing, striking in that : quite a group of remedies have produced hardness, soreness and tenderness of the gland; it may be one of those, or it may be one which has never produced these things, if it have the characterizing features of the patient.

In sickness the symptoms that cannot be explained are often very peculiar; the things that can be a accounted for are not so often peculiar: peculiar things are less known to man. For instance, a patient can sit only with his feet up on the desk, or with his feet elevated: he is a great sufferer, and because of this suffering he is compelled to put his feet up. The symptoms hence will be put down, worse from letting the feet hand down. "Well, what do you mean by that? Why, if I let my feet hang down, I find I bring the nates down upon the chair, and there is a sore place there." Now that is quite a different thing. You may find if it is an old man that he has a large prostate gland, which is very painful at times and very sore, and when he lets the feet hang down the gland comes in contact with the chair. So we see that the real summing up of the case is that this enlarged and sore prostate gland is worse from pressure, and all you have learned from that symptom is that the gland is sensitive to touch, which is a common symptom. There are instances, however, where by letting the feet hand down the patient in ameliorated; for instance, you take a periostitis and the pain is relieved by letting the limbs hang. No one can tell why that limb is better when hanging over the bed. He lies across the bed with the foot hanging over the side, and why it is that he cannot lie upon his back nobody can figure out. Now that condition is found in *Conium maculatum,* and you will not be astonished after you know that *Conium maculatum* has that symptom to find all the symptoms of your patient, say *Conium maculatum*. All the rest of them perhaps, are common.

Now, when you think along this line of science, it will not take you long to get into the habit of estimating among the symptoms that appear in a record the things that are common, the things that you would expect, and the things that are strange.

Again, we see that there are certain symptoms in the remedies that are *general* and on the other hand the symptoms that are general must also be taken into account in order to examine any record. All the things that are predicated of the patient himself are things that are general; all the things that are predicated of any given organ are things in particular. So we see how there are things in general, and things common, and things particular; sometimes it may be a condition or state, sometimes it may be a symptom. We have said that what the patient predicates of himself will generally appear to you to be at once something in general. When the patient says, "I am thirsty," as a matter of fact, although he feels that thirst in the mouth, yet it is his whole economy that craves the water.

The things of which he says, "I feel," are apt to be generals. The patient says, "I have so much burning," and if you examine him, you find that his head burns, that the skin burns, that there is burning in the anus, burning in the urine, and whatever region is affected burns. You find the word burning is a general feature that modifies all his sickness. If it were only in one organ, it would be a particular, but these things that relate to the whole of the man are things in general.

Again, when the patient tells things of his affections, he gives us things that are most general. When he speaks of his desires and aversions, we have those things that relate so closely to the man himself that the changes in these things will be marked by changes in his very ultimates. When the man arrives at that state that he has an aversion to life, we see that, that is a general symptom and that permeates his economy; that symptom qualifies all the symptoms and is the very center of all his states and conditions. When he has a desire to commit suicide, which is the loss of the love of his life, we see that that is very innermost, medicines affect man primarily by disturbing his affections, by disturbing his aversions and desires. The things that he loved to do are changed, and now he craves strange things. Or the remedy changes his ability to comprehend, and turns his life into a state of contention and disturbance; it disturbs his will and may bring upon him troublesome dreams, which are really mental states. Dreams are so closely allied to the mental state that he may well say, "I dreamed last night;" that is a general state. The things that lie closest to man and his life, and his vital force, are the things that are strictly general, and as they become less intimately related to man they become less and less general, until they become particular.

The menstrual period gives us a state, which we may call general. The woman says, "I menstruate," so and so; she does not attribute it to her ovaries or to her uterus; her state is, as a rule, different when she is menstruating. So the things that are predicated of self of the *ego,* the things described as "I do so and so," "Dr., I feel so and so," "I have so much thirst," "I am so chilly in every change of the weather," "I suffocate in a warm room," etc. these are all general. The things that are general are the first in importance. After these have been gathered, you may go on taking up each organ, and ascertaining what is true of each organ. Many times you will find that the modalities of each organ. Many times you will find that the modalities of each organ conform to the generals. Sometimes, however, there may be modalities of the organs, which are particular that are opposed to the general. Hence we find in remedies that appear to have in one subject one thing, and in another subject the very opposite of that thing. In one it will be a general, and in another it will be a particular.

Classroom Notes

The Value of Symptoms

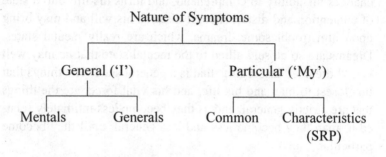

Nature of Symptoms

General ('I')   Particular ('My')

Mentals   Generals   Common   Characteristics
                                                    (SRP)

1. General symptoms, where the Patient says "*I feel*".

2. Particular symptoms, where the patient says "*my part feels*".

3. Common symptoms are diagnostic of disease.

4. Characteristic symptoms are diagnostic of the individual suffering from disease. These are also called the strange, rare or peculiar symptoms (SRP).

5. It is the peculiar way in which the same disease affects different patient with different symptoms. This individuality makes the symptom *strange, rare and peculiar*.

6. That which is *pathognomic* in the remedy is the thing you will study the most, because it is related to the patient. Such is the state of mind that the Homeopathic physician must keep in order to begin this study and cure patients.

7. Now when you think along this line of science, it will not take you long to get into the habit of estimating the symptoms that appear in your record as the things that are common, the things that you will expect and the things that are strange.

8. When you begin to think in this way then you can study symptoms of the disease as 'Grade'.

9. Symptoms are:

a) Recorded (in provings).

b) Confirmed (by reprovings).

c) Verified (by clinical use on the sick).

10. **Grades of symptoms** (as used in Kent's repertory):

   (a) **Grade I:** Symptoms that are proved, confirmed and verified.

   (b) **Grade II:** Symptoms that are proved on some provers but have been confirmed and sometimes verified.

   (c) **Grade III:** Prover have brought out a symptom, which has not been confirmed but has been verified clinically by some.

LECTURE XXXIII

The Value of Symptoms (Continued)

IT is very important that you should understand what is meant by general, common and particular symptoms and so I will repeat somewhat. The generals are sometimes made up of particulars. If you examine any part alone, you are only examining the particulars. If you examine the liver symptoms alone, you are examining particulars. If you are examining the eye symptoms, or the symptoms of any other region considered apart from the whole man, you are examining particular symptoms. But after you have gathered the particulars of every region of the body, and you see there are certain symptoms running through the particulars, those symptoms that run through the particulars have become generals, as well as particulars.

Things that apply to all the organs may be predicated of the person himself. Things that modify all parts of the organism are those that relate to the general state. Anything that the individual predicates of himself is also general. There are things that an individual might say of himself that might relate to only one organ, but of course of that becomes a particular; but most of the things that the man predicates of himself are general.

Consider for instance, the symptoms of sleep. You might at first think that they relate to the brain, but the brain does not sleep any more than the whole man. "I was wakeful last night;" he is predicating something of himself and hence it is a general. Or, he says, "I dreamed;" well it is true that the whole man really dreamed. You might say that the mind merely dreamed, but the mind is the man, and therefore, we see how important sleep and dreams become in the anamnesis of a case. Scarcely more important is what the women says of her menstruation; menstruation so closely relates to the whole women that it becomes most important. The special senses also are so closely related to the whole man that the smells that are grateful and the smells that are disagreeable become general.

There are certain smells that relate more particularly to the nose itself, because the smell is in the nose and is due to some pathological condition of the nose, and thus becomes a mere particular. The smell of food is agreeable when the man is hungry, and that will relate to the whole man, but one who has a vicious catarrh of the nose, with much local disturbance, has many perversions of smell, which are particular, because they relate to the nose. A patient says: "I see" so and so, without seeing; that relates to the generals. It is to great extent a seeing with the understanding. Now, when the eye itself becomes affected, the symptoms gathered are particulars because they relate to the anatomy of the eye. The more the symptoms relate to the anatomy of the parts, the more external they are : the more they relate to the tissues, the more likely they are to be particular. But the more they relate to internals that involve the whole man, the more they become general.

The things, therefore, that relate to the man are the ones to be singled our in the anamnesis and marked first. After gathering together all the symptoms of a patient you should single out for study first of all everything and anything that you can predicate of the man, everything of which you can say *he* feels so and so, *she* suffers so and so. Find out what remedies relate to these symptoms first. Sometimes when you have figured the anamnesis of the generals, you have settled by your anamnesis upon three remedies, or possibly upon one. In ninety-nine cases of a hundred you can leave out the particulars, for the particulars are usually contained within the general, and covers those generals absolutely and clearly and strongly, that will be the remedy that will cure the case. There may be a lot of little particulars that may appear to contra-indicate, but they cannot; for nothing in particulars can contra-indicate generals. One strong general can over rule all the particulars you can gather up. "Aggravation from heat" will throw out *Arsenicum album* from consideration in any case.

It may be advisable to dwell again for a little upon the common symptoms. Sometimes we find in woman the *common* symptom, prolapsus. It is a common thing for them to say, "Doctor, I have such a dragging down in my bowels, as if my insides were coming out." That is a common feature, and it is a common symptom. There is nothing about that alone that will enable you to find a remedy, but for these common symptoms we have a class of remedies. When you see a rubric containing a dozen, fifteen or twenty remedies, you may often know it is a common symptom. We would say that all women who have prolapsus have to a great extent a dragging down feeling, as if the uterus would come out. If we were to take this symptom and follow it up, we would see that it works in various directions; we would see that it runs into generals, and into particulars. How shall we decide when to give *Sep.*, when *Lil-t.*, when *Murex*, when *Bell.*, when *Puls.*, when *Nux vomica*, and when *Natrium muriaticum?* To enable you to pick out of that group of remedies the one that will cure you must study both the generals and the particulars of the patient and the generals always first. If it be a *Nux vomica* patient who has the prolapsus of the uterus, what will she say of herself that will make you see *Nux vomica* in it? She would be chilly; full of coryza, with stuffing up of the nose in a warm room; she would be very irritable, snappish, want to kill somebody, want to throw her child into the fire, want to kill her husband. She would probably have constipation and every pain she had with it would make her want to go to stool; urging to stool but only a little is passed and she wants to go frequently. You see at once that she has the generals of *Nux vomica*, and whatever particulars she has are in harmony with those generals, and so you go from generals to particulars. The whole problem, like any other scientific problem, must be gone into and followed from generals to particulars. Suppose that *Sepia officinalis* is indicated for that women. You have in it as well this common symptom. Now, what is there in this patient that no other patient has? The dragging down is just the same, but with it an awful all-gone sinking feeling in the stomach, and she gets relief only when sitting with the legs crossed. She has a constant feeling of a lump in the rectum that makes her want to go to stool, but she goes for days without any urging at all; she is sallow and sickly, talks of bilious symptoms and has a yellow saddle over the nose. She tells that she has an aversion to her children, and feels very sad that she does not love her husband as she ought to. She is unable to exercise the love she has to her children. Now you have that which she says of herself in general, and that which she tells of the stomach and rectum in particular, and yet peculiar. You can see now that the dragging down sensation is not general nor particular, but is common.

Many of the symptoms of regions are both common and particular, particular because they are of regions and common because they describe a state. Scarlet fever gives us an illustration of this. We would group all the striking symptoms indicative of scarlet fever, the rash, the appearance of the mucous membranes, the sore throat, the fever, the history, and the period of prodrome. The remedies for scarlet fever must have these symptoms in common with scarlet fever. The appearance of scarlet fever is among the common things of *Belladonna. Ailanthus glandulosa* has in its common things the appearance of scarlet fever; *Apis* has the appearance of rough scarlet fever. *Sulphur* and *Phosphorus* have a rash similar to scarlet fever. So if we were to make a rubric for the repertory we would put the names of all these remedies in the common group and call it scarlet fever.

But when are you going to give one remedy and when another? We can sometimes figure our from local manifestations thing in general. For instance, you can take an *Arum triphyllum* patient; that which appears to be most striking is that he picks his nose and lips until they bleed. If you examine that state well you will ascertain that these parts and the fingers and toes tingle; about the extremities where the circulation is feeble and where the nerves are abundant, in the nerves of the fingres and toes, there is an unusual tingling like the creeping of ants, and he keeps picking at these parts. It is a state marking almost the whole economy. If you watch a little more closely, you will see that liquid oozes out of the parts he has picked, a bloody, watery oozing, and that it denudes the skin around the parts. It becomes a part of the general state. Then in scarlet fever, with the rash only partly out, we want to take the language of nature alone. I spoke of *Phosphorus.* *Phos.* has a typical scarlet fever rash. Suppose you have a case that is putrid, the rash has become very dusky and the skin has become mottled and purplish, and there are places about the body that have a tendency to suppurate. You find there are swellings about the neck, swellings upon the hands and fingers, that are inclined to suppurate; or there is an oozing round about them and pus is welling forth, and the case is so putrid and offensive that as soon as you enter the room you detect the horrible stench, if you examine into the case, you will see that the child cannot get water enough and cannot get it cold enough. The countenance is sunken, and the eyes are puffed and swollen and red. Blotches are appearing of a specific character intermingled with the scarlet fever blotches. There you have a *Phos.* case, and *Phos.* will stop the trouble immediately. Now, what have you gathered together? You have gathered together an evidence of the general state. You see running all through that case putridity and a zymotic state. You may have many cases of malignant scarlet fever, and you will find that you can manage them with your remedies as you would an unruly horse with reins.

Now as to the grades. The value of symptoms is divided into three grades. General symptoms are divided into three grades, first, second and third, and common symptoms and particular symptoms are divided into the same three grades. You will see in Bœnninghausen a fourth grade, but as a matter of fact these remedies do not form a grade, they are only probationary remedies, requiring demonstration by reproving and clinical confirmation.

The general symptoms of the first grade are such as all or the majority of provers state of themselves as a class of provers. For instance, take that symptom of *Apis,* " suffocation in a warm room;" all the provers of *Apis,* or nearly all were affected to a great extent in that way. All the provers of *Pulsatilla nigricans* were worse in a warm room. There can be no doubt about such symptoms for all the provers felt that state so strongly. *Kali-i., Pulsatilla, Iodium* and *Apis* are among those that have that symptom in the first grade, worse in a warm room, suffocation in a warm room. Now when those symptoms which have existed as generals among the provers come into the experience of the practitioner, and are confirmed by curing those states extensively, wherever administered, for years, then these remedies are fully entitled to this grade. When only one prover has recorded a certain symptom, it is doubtful whether that is a symptom from the action of the remedy, but when several provers have recorded the same symptom it becomes confirmed. When that symptom has been removed or cured by the remedy in the hands of a physician, it can then be said to have been verified. So symptoms are (1) recorded, (2) confirmed by reprovings, and (3) verified upon the sick. When several provers have observed that *Puls.* is worse in a warm room, and this is confirmed by other provers, and then verified by cure upon the sick, it immediately places *Pulsatilla nigricans* in the first grade of that general state. Suppose that it were something that was in relation to the bladder; *Puls.* as a symptom of frequent urination; now, that is immediately classified as a particular symptom because it relates to a region. Now, if all of these provers had irritable bladder when they took *Puls.* that would be a confirmation of it, and if it cures for years experience verifies it and it is then placed as belonging to *Pulsatilla nigricans* under the particulars, and marked in the highest grade. So with the symptom of bearing down, which also comes under *Pulsatilla nigricans;* that would be classed as a common symptom, but of the first grade.

Suppose now that there are more symptoms that have only been brought out by a few of the provers; they do not run through the whole family of provers, but they have been confirmed and occasionally verified; then you see they are not entitled to so much consideration and as a matter of degree they belong to the *second* grade, because not so strong as the first grade, which produces these symptoms upon everybody or nearly everybody. Of course, what is true of the generals will be true of common and particular. Then as to the *third* grade. Now and then a prover brings out a symptom and it has not yet been confirmed by reproving, but it stands out pretty strong, and seems to be worthy of a third place, or it has been verified by having cured sick folks, or on the other hand it is admitted as a clinical symptom. Sometimes close and careful observers have noticed that certain symptoms, not in the proving, have generally yielded to a certain remedy, and others have confirmed this clinical experience; these symptoms are admitted to go into the third grade. A great many of Bœnninghausen's fourth grade symptoms really belong to the third grade, because Bœnninghausen was very cautious with the symptoms that had never been verified. His fourth grade remedies include such as he had gathered from his clinical experience, and he was doubtful about the propriety of placing them in the third grade, and also those symptoms that occurred in the provers but had not proper confirmation or were not verified. He laid them, as it were, upon a shelf for approbation, to be hereafter proved or accepted.

LECTURE XXXIV

The Homoeopathic Aggravation

§ 154 (LAST clause). "A disease that is of no very long standing ordinarily yields without any great degree of suffering to the first dose of this remedy," which is to say that in acute disease we seldom see anything like striking aggravation unless the acute disease has drawn near death's door, or is very severe, unless it has lasted many days, and breaking down of blood and tissue is threatened or has taken place. Then we will see sharp aggravations, great prostration, violent sweating, exhaustion, vomiting and purging following the action of the remedy. I have seen most severe reaction which seemed to be necessary to recovery. Such a state in acute disease where it has gone many days without a remedy and a great threatening is present will be to an acute disease what many years would be to a chronic disease of long standing. Long standing means as a matter of progress; if we say a disease of much progress, or of considerable ultimates, we understand it better. If the disease has ultimated itself in change of tissue, then you see striking aggravations, even aggravations that cannot be recovered from, such as we find in the advanced forms of tissue change, e.g., where the kidneys are destroyed or the liver destroyed, or in phthisis, where the lungs are destroyed.

A disease ought always to be well considered as to whether it is acute or chronic. Where there are no tissue changes, where no ultimates are present, then you may expect the remedy to cure the patient without any serious aggravation, or without any sharp suffering, for there is no necessity of reacting from a serious structural change. Where there is a deep-seated septic condition, where pyaemia must be the result, you will find sometimes vomiting and purging. As a reaction of the vital force of the economy when order is established, this order, which is attended by reaction, as it were commences a process of house cleaning. It does it itself, the drug does not do it; if a crude substance is used it is the action of the drug, of course, but the action of the dynamic drug is to turn the economy into order. So it is with chronic disease. When the chronic disease has not ultimated itself in tissue changes, you may get no aggravation at all, unless, perhaps, it be a very slight exacerbation of the symptoms, and that slight exacerbation of the symptoms is of a different character. It is the establishment of the remedy as a new disease upon the economy instead of the reaction, which corresponds to a process of house cleaning. Elimination must take place, as we know, probably from the bowels, or stomach, by vomiting, by expectoration, or by the kidneys, in those cases where everything has been suppressed.

It may look like an aggravation when you have had for years a limb paralyzed from a neuritis. Suppose, after you administer a remedy that goes right to the spot, that is in the very highest sense homoeopathic, or truly specific, that paralyzed limb commences to tingle and creep like the crawling interiorly of ants, tingling sometimes from which he cannot sleep for days and nights. This is due to the reaction of the nerves of the part. They are called into new life, into activity. I have seen this in paralysis. You take, for instance, a child who has 'lain' in a stupor for a long time, from inaction of the brain, the tingling that comes in the scalp, in the fingers and toes is dreadful, the child turns and twists and screeches and cries, and it requires an iron hand on the part of the doctor to hold that mother from doing something to hush that cry, for just so sure as that is done that child will go back into death. That is a reaction, so that all over the benumbed parts, or where the blood begins to flow into parts where the circulation has been feeble, where the nerves take on sensation again, we have reaction; which is but the result of that turning into order. That part has been benumbed and dead, and when circulation takes place in the part in order to repair its tissue we have reaction, which is attended with distress. If the physician cannot look upon that and bear it, he will have trouble. If he thinks it is an indication for another remedy he will spoil his case.

We must discriminate between that which is reaction and that which calls for a remedy. These things are only seen in homoeopathy, never in any practice. Sometimes the physician will be driven to his wit's end in dealing with these reactions. It is sometimes in a dreadful thing to look upon, and the physician may be turned out of doors. Let him meet it as a man; let him be patient with it, because the ignorance of the mother or the friends can be no excuse for his violation of principle, even once.

A disease of very long standing sometimes fails to yield without this aggravation and disturbance and turmoil in the economy, and the deeper it is the more tissue change you have to contend with, and the more wonderful and distressing and painful is this reaction. When a patient comes back after every dose of medicine with violent reaction, with violent aggravation of the disease, with violent aggravation of the symptoms, you know then that there is some deep-seated trouble. There is a difference between the ultimates of disease and absolute weakness of the vital force. There is such a state as weakness of the economy, and there is such a state as activity of the economy, with much tissue change. In feeble patients you may expect feeble reactions, or none at all after your remedy, but in the feeble cases they are of such character that you have few symptoms, and you can very seldom find a remedy truly specific.

For example, say you get a patient that is destined to go into consumption, a merely suspicious case. You administer the right remedy and a violent reaction comes, a foreshadowing of what he will go through years from now if he is not cured by the remedy. A shocking condition will come upon him; he may be frightened and come back and tell you that, that was an awful dose of medicine, poison, etc. That is the remedy disease, those are the symptoms of the remedy foreshadowing the future of that case, because if that remedy was not similar enough to him it could not do such things, and it is because of the similitude of his state; and he may only have those symptoms in shadow. But the remedy cannot give him symptoms that he has not. It cannot give him symptoms that are not related to him except in those cases that are called oversensitives. Oversensitives, you know are such as are capable of proving everything that comes along. You must know whether the patient is oversensitive and proving the drug, or whether he has a vigorous constitution and is getting an aggravation. The remedy will be exaggerated in oversensitives and sometimes in those of weakly constitution, especially those with a very narrow receding chin, those who have sunken eyes, those who have senility marked in the eyes.

The next paragraph continues this one to a certain extent. Par. 155. "I say without any degree of suffering, because when a perfect homoeopathic remedy acts upon the body, it is nothing more than symptoms analogous to those of the disease laboring to surmount and annihilate these latter by usurping their place." This is only speaking from experience. Whenever Hahnemann makes such a remark he does not place any great value upon it, because it is a matter of opinion.

You will find as a general thing in acute diseases, that if a slight aggravation of the symptoms comes in a few minutes, you will hardly ever think of giving another dose. The remedy is so similar and searches so thoroughly that it is hardly ever necessary to repeat it. Now there are circumstances when it is necessary to repeat, but this is so difficult to teach, and so difficult to lay down rules for, that the only safe plan is to begin cases without repetition, to give a single dose and wait, and watch its effects. I very commonly give in vigorous, typhoid fever patients medicines in water, because it is a continued fever; but I watch and wait, giving it several days, and the slightest sign of the action of the remedy causes me to stop it always. I never vary from that. In a fever where the patient is feeble, to gain an immediate reaction that should never be done.

In a remittent fever the reaction may come in a very few hours, and the one dose should be the rule, while in a typhoid the reaction will seldom come in a few hours. It is matter of a few days, and hence the repetition is admissible. In typhoids that are somewhat delicate never do such a thing? The more vigor there is in a constitution the more the remedy can co-operate with that vigor to bring about a safe and quick action.

The more feeble the patient the more cautious you should be about using the smallest dose you can give. In many chronic disease it is possible to bring about a reaction in the first night, hence the danger of repeating the remedy. If the delirium subsides, or a moisture comes upon the skin, and he slumbers placidly, the medicine should never be given beyond such a state. There are times in diphtheria when the repetition of the remedy will kill, and there are times when repetition will safe life. I hope some day to be able to discover the principles.

§ 158. "This trifling homoeopathic aggravation of the malady during the first few hours, the happy omen which announces that the acute disease will soon be cured, and that it will, for the most part, yield to a first dose." That a natural disease can destroy another by exceeding it in power and intensity, but above all things by its similarity, is the whole truth and nothing but the truth. So that when this slight aggravation occurs you will seldom, if ever, have to give another dose in an acute disease. When this aggravation does not come, when there is not the slightest aggravation of the symptoms, and the patient appears to be gradually better after the remedy, then it is that the remedy shows that it has not acted upon the same depth; and that relief ceases in the case of an acute disease, and when that relief ceases the reaction has ceased and then another dose of medicine is correct practice.

Relief that begins without any aggravation of the symptoms does not last so long in an acute disease as when an aggravation has taken place. A slight action of the remedy over and above the disease is a good sign. Again, you will find if your remedy was not perfectly similar you will not get an aggravation except in over sensitive patients, and then it is a medicinal aggravation. When you find that you get no aggravation or the symptoms in a good vigorous constitution, none at all, very often your remedy has been only partially similar and it may require two or three of such partially similar remedies to finish the case. If you will observe the work of ordinary physicians, you will notice they give two or three remedies to finish the case. If you will observe the work of ordinary physician, you will notice they give two or three remedies to get their patients through where a master gives but one.

§ 159. "The smaller the dose of the homoeopathic remedy, the slighter the apparent aggravation of the disease, and it is proportionately of shorter duration." This was written at the time of Hahnemann's experience with what might be called small doses, ranging from the lower potencies to the 30th and seldom much higher. He had had ample experience with the 30th, and occasionally with the 60th, but not with tremendous turmoil that comes from the very highest attenuations. It reads in the correct translation of it (this is incorrect here) : "The smaller the dose is of the homoeopathic medicine, the less and the shorter is the aggravation in the first hours." It might be considered to mean an apparent aggravation, or an apparent aggravation of the disease. Now Hahnemann observes, as you will find amongst several of his writings, that the disease itself is actually intensified and made worse by the remedy, if the remedy be precisely similar, but if we pass away from the crudity of the medicines, ranging up towards the 30th potency, we get a milder action, and it has a deeper curative action, and the smaller the dose of the homoeopathic medicine the less and the shorter is the aggravation. The idea is that there is an aggravation in the first hours; that is a matter that the paragraph itself admits, and it is this aggravation that Hahnemann is talking about.

It is sometimes true that after the third or fourth potencies of *Belladonna* in a violent congestion of the brain, the aggravation is violent, and if the medicine is not discontinued the child will die. The disease itself appears to be aggravated, the child seems to be so susceptible to Belladonna that it appears as it were to be added to the disease, but with the 30th potency, as Hahnemann observes, this aggravation is slight and of short duration. Now, in this we get an outside aggravation. It is the drug disease of the remedy added to the natural disease, an aggravated state of the disease caused by the drug. It is true sometimes, in spite of this aggravation, that the patient says somehow or other he feels better.

This aggravation is unnecessarily prolonged by giving too low potencies; it is also prolonged by a repetition of the dose. I recently observed a state that occurred from repetition. I sent a very robust young woman, twenty years old, a dose of *Bryonia alba*, to be taken dry on the tongue. However, she dissolved it in water, and was taking it at the end of the second day, when I was sent for, at which time she seemed to be going into pneumonia. She had a dry, harsh cough. "What is the matter with my daughter, doctor, is she the going to die?" She was proving Bryonia. I stopped the *Bryonia alba*, and next morning she was well. This has been seen a great many times when the medicine was similar. If the medicine is not very similar, only partially similar it yet may be similar enough to cure, but you will not see the results that I am now speaking of; but when you make accurate prescriptions, and are doing your best work, you will see these things in the very best constitutions.

Of course, the explanation is that the patient is as sensitive to the medicine that will cure her as to the disease that she has. Diseased states, then, are made worse by unnecessary repetition and by the dose not being small enough, that is, by the dose being very crude. The third, fourth and sixth are dangerous potencies, if you are a good prescriber. If you are a poor prescriber, you will demonstrate but little of anything. You will naturally go to the higher and higher potencies for the purpose of departing from what seems to be poisonous dose.

This action differs from the aggravation of a c.m potency, during the latter the patient feels decidedly better. It is short, it is decisive, and only the characteristic symptoms of the disease are aggravated. The disease itself is not aggravated; the disease itself is not added to, and is not intensified, but the symptoms of the disease stand out sharply and the patient says, "I am getting better." The symptoms sometimes are a little alarming, but intermingled with this is a ray of light that convinces the patient from his innermost feelings that he is getting better. "I feel much better this morning," says the patient, though the symptoms may have been sharpened up.

§ 160. We are accused nowadays of having departed from Hahnemann . Hahnemann wrote of the 30th potency in one of the stages of his life, as sufficiently high and sufficiently low. We can easily see that it was in the earlier period of his investigations that he made the remark that potentizing must end somewhere. We are accused of departing from Hahnemann, because we give different doses from what Hahnemann gave. Now I want to show you that this is not so. Read paragraph 279: "It has been fully proved by pure experiments that when a disease does not evidently depend upon the impaired state of an important organ *the dose of the homoeopathic remedy can never be sufficiently small so as to be inferior to the power of the natural disease which it can, at least, partially extinguish and cure, provided it be capable of producing only a small increase of symptoms immediately after it is administered"* Now, if we go to the 200th potency and find that they will aggravate, if we go to the 50m. and find that that will aggravate, if we go to the cm., the mm., etc., and find that they will aggravate, that they still have the power to intensify the symptoms, the remedy has just the same curative power in it. If we have the potency so high that it is not capable of producing an aggravation of the symptoms, we may then be sure that there is no medicinal power left. We are up to the 13mm. and the end is not yet.

Now we have never made the claim that every potency will suit everybody. The potency must correspond to the state of the patient. If we ever find a person who will be aggravated in his symptoms in the most positive and definite fashion, that potency will be verified. We have departed from Hahnemann, but have acted in accordance with his doctrines. § 280. "This incontrovertible axiom, founded upon experience will serve as a rule by which the doses of all homoeopathic medicines, without exception, are to be attenuated to such a degree, that after being introduced into the body they shall merely produce an almost insensible aggravation of the disease. It is of little importance whether the attenuation goes so far as to appear almost impossible to ordinary physicians whose minds feed on no other ideas but are gross and material. All these arguments and vain assertions will be if little avail when opposed to the doctrines of unerring experience."

Now, can there be any doubt of what Hahnemann meant when he speaks of the smallest dose? Can there be any doubt but that he means attenuation, attenuation up and up until we reach that point in the attenuation that we do not observe a slight aggravation of the symptoms ? In the note to paragraph 249; he says, "All experience teaches us that scarcely any homoeopathic medicine can be prepared in too minute a dose to produce perceptible benefit in a disease to which it is adapted. Hence, it would be an improper and an injurious practice when the medicine produces no good effect or an inconsiderable aggravation of the symptoms, after the manner of the old school to repeat or increase the dose under the ideas that it cannot prove serviceable on account of its minuteness."

So the senses have no relation whatever to the minuteness of the dose. The medical man is inclined to measure doses from the standard of a poisonous dose. He will measure off a little less than that which would poison, and call that a dose. It must be seen, it must yet be visible. This is not the test that Hahnemann offers. He offers the test of the dose as one capable of producing a slight aggravation of the symptoms. We see he does not limit attenuation, but he practically teaches it is unlimited, and the end has never been found.

There is a generally prevailing idea all over, not among strict Hahnemannians, but among modern homeopaths in general, that the dose of medicine laid down by Hahnemann is too small to cure. It is a fatal error. An increase of the dose cannot make it more homoeopathic. The similarity of the remedy is first, and the dose is second. But that the dose of medicine laid down by Hahnemann is too small to cure is a fatal error. We must see by the experience in the clinics, and by considering the wonderful things that we have gone over in the doctrines, that we have really very little to do with the dose, that there is a wonderful latitude in dosage, and that we cannot lay down any fixed rule as to the best potency to use.

It ought to be distinctly felt, from all we have gone over, that the 30th potency is low enough to begin business with in any acute or chronic disease, but where the limit is no mortal can see. We want to follow up the series, so that we may get the internal states that exist in degrees in the medicine. The different potencies are distinct from each other, some are very far apart, yet invariably connected. It is a mistake for any homœopath to start out with the idea that the dose of medicine laid down by Hahnemann is too small to cure. It shows that his mind is of material mould, that it is inelastic and cannot yield to the higher observations, and not capable of observing and following higher and higher as true experience would lead. Unless man has truth in his mind his experiences are false. Truth in the mind is first and then experiences are good. If his mind is in a state of truth, experiences are true. You cannot trust the experiences of men who do not know what is true, neither can they be led into truth by these fallacious experiences.

Classroom Notes

The Homeopathic Aggravation

1. If the disease has resulted itself in change of tissues, then you see striking aggravation (even aggravation that cannot be recovered from) such as seen in advanced destructive pathologies of lung, liver, kidney etc. If chronic disease has not resulted itself in tissue changes, you may see no aggravation at all, unless perhaps, it be a very light exacerbation of the symptoms.

2. Aggravation is of two kinds:

(a) *Aggravation of disease*, in which the patient is growing worse.

(b) *Aggravation of symptoms*, in which the patient is growing better.

3. Another exacerbation is like house cleaning which is not an aggravation by definition. It is an *Elimination*. This elimination might take place as *diarrhea, vomiting, perspiration, expectoration, urination* or *eruption of a rash*.

4. If a patient comes back after every dose of medicine with violent reaction, with violent aggravation of disease you know that there is some deep seated trouble which can be one of the following:

(a) This patient is an oversensitive one and proves any and everything that is given to him.

(b) If this aggravation is prolonged then the patient is of feeble constitution with advanced disease.

(c) If the aggravation is sharp and short, then the patient is of robust constitution.

5. The more feeble the patient the more cautions you must be. Use the smallest dose you can give.

6. A safe plan is to begin cases without repetition (specially when using high potencies). Give a dose then wait and watch.

7. If signs and actions of remedy appear then stop, do not interfere till relief is reported.

8. When relief ceases, the reaction has ceased and another dose of medicine is needed.

9. If relief begins without any aggravation of symptoms (specially in acute disease) then it does not last as long as when an aggravation would have taken place.

10. When you find that you get no aggravation of symptoms in a good vigorous constitution; none at all, very often your remedy has been only partially similar and it may require two or three of such similar remedies to finish the case.

[Para: 159]

The smaller the dose of the Homeopathic remedy the slighter the apparent aggravation of the disease and it is proportionately of shorter duration.

1. As we pass away from the crudity of medicine i.e. mother tincture to 30C and beyond we get milder action, and it has deeper curative action.
2. The idea is that, an aggravation occurs in first few hours.
3. This aggravation is unnecessarily prolonged by going too low in potencies and also prolonged by unnecessary repetition of the dose.
4. The 3C, 4C, 6C are dangerous potencies for a good prescriber.
5. The initial aggravation of higher potencies is different. This aggravation is short and decisive and only the characteristic symptoms of the disease are aggravated. The disease itself is not aggravated. Disease is not added to, it is not intensified but symptoms of disease stand out sharply while the patient says 'I am getting better'.

[Para: 160 also 279, 280, 249]

1. The similarity of the remedy is the first requisite and potency is the second.
2. The same potency will not suit everybody. Potency must be carefully selected. It must correspond to the state of the patient and to the plane of disease.
3. It is a mistake for any Homeopath to start with the idea, that the dose of medicine laid down by Hahnemann, is too small to cure.
4. In Para 279, Hahnemann does not limit attenuation but he practically teaches that it is unlimited and the end has never been found.
5. It must be distinctively perceived that 30 C is low enough to begin business with any acute or chronic disease.

LECTURE XXXV

Prognosis after Observing the Action of the Remedy

AFTER a prescription has been made the physician commences to make observations. The whole future of the patient may depend upon the conclusions that the physician arrives at from these observations, for his action depends very much upon his observations, and upon his action depends the good of the patient. If he is not conversant with the import of what he sees, he will undertake to do wrong things, he will make wrong prescriptions, he will change his medicines and do things to the detriment of the patient. There is absolutely but one way, and nothing can take the place of intelligence. If you talk with a great many physicians concerning the observations you have made after giving the remedy you will find that the majority of them have only whims or notions on this subject and see nothing after the prescription is made. These observations I am going to give you have grown out of much watchfulness, long waiting and watching. If the homoeopathic physician is not an accurate observer, his observations will be indefinite; and if his observations are indefinite, his prescribing is indefinite.

It is taken for granted after a prescription has been made, and it is an accurate prescription, that it has acted. Now, if a medicine is acting it commences immediately to affect changes in the patient, and these changes are shown by signs and symptoms. The inner nature of the disease appears to the physician through the symptoms, and it is like watching the hands upon the clock. This watching and waiting and observing has to be done by the physician in order that he may judge by the changes what to do, and what not to do. It is true that the homœopath is not long in doubt in many instances what not to do. There is always an index that tells him what not to do. If he is a sharp and vigilant observer, he will see the index for every case. Of course, if a prescription is not related to the case, if it is a prescription that effects no changes, it does not take long to see what to do; much patient waiting for a foolish prescription is but loss of time, and that should be taken into account among the observations. The observations taken after a specific remedy has been given sufficiently related to the case to cause changes in the symptoms are those of value.

The changes are beginning, what are they like, what do they mean, to what do they amount? The physician must know when he listens to the reports of the patient what is going on. The remedy is known to act by the changing of the symptoms. The disappearance of symptoms, the increase of symptoms, the amelioration of symptoms, the order of the symptoms, are all changes from the remedy, and these changes are to be studies.

Among the commonest things that remedies do is to aggravate or ameliorate. The aggravation is of two kinds; we may have an aggravation, which is an aggravation of the disease, in which the patient is growing worse, or we may have an aggravation of the symptoms, in which the patient is growing better. An aggravation of the disease means that the patient is growing weaker, the symptoms are growing stronger; but the homoeopathic aggravation, which is the aggravation of the symptoms of the patient while the patient is growing better, is something that the physician observes, after a true homoeopathic prescription. The true homoeopathic aggravation, I say, is when the symptoms are worse, but the patient says, "I feel better."

We must now go into the particulars concerning these states, as to the time and place, as to how the aggravation occurs, as to how the amelioration occurs, as to duration, etc. The aggravations and ameliorations, the direction of symptoms and many other things have to come up, and be observed and judgement has to be passed upon them.

First of all the patient should be the aim of the physician, his whole idea should be centered upon the patient to determine whether he is improving or declining. We have to judge by the symptoms to know that this is taking place. Very often the patient will say, "I am growing weaker," and yet you may know that what he says is not true; so certainly can you rely upon the symptoms and their story, which is more faithful than the patient's opinion. Many times the patient will say, "Doctor, I am so much worse;" and yet you examine into his symptoms and you find that he is really doing very well. Just the moment that he finds out that you are encouraged, he feels better and rouses up and wants to eat.

By the symptoms, also, you can tell when the patient is really weaker, and if the symptoms are taking an inward rather than an outward course you will know, even if he is encouraged, that there is no encouragement for him. We have in the symptoms that which we can rely upon. In the old school we have nothing but the information of the patient. This is of little account after making a homoeopathic prescription. The symptoms themselves must be corroborated. The patient's opinion must be corroborated by the symptoms. The symptoms do corroborate what the patients say in many instances, but the symptoms are the physician's most satisfactory evidence.

Another general remark needs to be made, namely, that we should know by the symptoms if the changes occurring are sufficiently interior. If the changes that are occurring are exterior, the physician must be acquainted with the meaning of them, so that he will know by that whether the disease is being healed from the innermost or whether the symptoms have merely changed according to their superficial nature. Incurable diseases will very often be palliated by mild medicines that act only superficially, act upon the sensorium, act upon the sense, and, though the hidden and deep-seated trouble goes on and progresses, and is sometimes made worse, yet the patient is made comfortable. So that by the symptoms we can know whether the changes that are occurring are of sufficient depth, so that the patient may recover. The direction that the symptoms are taking is sufficient to tell that, especially in chronic disease.

A patient walks into the clinic, somewhat stoop-shouldered, with a hacking cough that he has had for a good many years. You judge by his looks that he has been sick a good while; his face is sickly, he is lean and anxious, he is careworn, he is suffering from poverty and poor clothing and scanty food. Now, you examine all of his symptoms, and they clearly indicate that he needs an antipsoric, for the symptoms are covered by an antipsoric, and from the history of the case you know he has needed it a good while. Upon prolonged examination, the antipsoric you have in mind is strengthened. You now examine his chest, and discover he has not the expansion that he ought to have, and you detect the presence of tuberculosis, and by feeble pulse and many other corroborating symptoms you ascertain that the patient has been steadily declining.

You give the medicine and he comes back in a few days with quite a sharp aggravation of the symptoms; he has an increased cough, he has a night sweat, and he is more feeble. Now, the homoeopathic physician likes to hear that; he likes to hear of an exacerbation of the symptoms; but this patient comes back in a week, and the aggravation is still present, and is somewhat on the increase, the patient is coughing worse, and the expectoration is more troublesome than ever, his night sweats have been going on; he comes back at the end of the second week and he is still worse, and all the symptoms have been worse since he took that medicine. He was comparatively comfortable before he took that medicine, but at the end of the fourth week he is steadily growing worse. There has been no amelioration following this aggravation, and he is evidently declining; he now cannot come to the office for he is so weak.

This, then, will be the *first observation - a prolonged aggravation and final decline of the patient.* What have we done? It has been a mistake, the antipsoric was too deep, it has established destruction. In this state the vital reaction was impossible, he was an incurable case. The question immediately comes up, what are you to do? Are you not going to give the homoeopathic remedy in such cases? The patient steadily declines. If you are in doubt about such action of the remedies and making the patient worse, you will probably have an undertaker's certificate to sign before long.

In incurable and doubtful cases give no higher than the 30th or 200th potency, and observe whether the aggravation is going to be too deep or too prolonged. There are many signs in the chest in such cases to make a physician doubt whether he will give a deep remedy when organic disease is present. Of course this does not apply when things are only threatening, when you have fear of their coming, but when you are sure of their being present. In the instance given the probability is that the remedy has been too late, and it has attempted to arouse his economy, but turned to destruction his whole organism. Then begin, in such cases with a moderately low potency, and the 30th is low enough for anybody or anything.

When the patient does not seem to be quite so bad as the one I have just described, you get him a little earlier in his history before the trouble has gone quite so far, and then if you administer this same very high potency in the same way you will make a second observation. Though the aggravation is long and severe, yet you have a final reaction, or amelioration. The aggravation lasts for many weeks, perhaps, and then his feeble economy seems to react, and there is a slow but sure improvement. It shows that the disease has not progressed quite so far; the changes have not become quite so marked. At the end of three months he is prepared for another does of medicine, and you see a repetition of the same thing, and you may know then that, that man was on the border land and had he gone further, cure would have been impossible. It is always well in doubtful cases to go to the lower potencies, and in this way go cautiously prepared to antidote the medicine if it takes the wrong course.

Then the *second observation* is, the *long aggravation, but final and slow improvement.* If, at the end of a few weeks, he is a little better and his symptoms are a little better than when he took the dose, there is some hope that finally the symptoms may have an outward manifestation whereby he will attain final recovery, but for many years you may go along with prolonged aggravations. You will find in such a patient there was the beginning of some very marked tissue change in some organ. We may know by observing the action, of a remedy what state the tissues are in, as well as know something about the prognosis for the patient.

The *third observation* after administering the homoeopathic remedy is, where the *aggravation is quick, short and strong with rapid improvement of the patient.* Whenever you find an aggravation comes quickly, is short, and has been more or less vigorous, then you will find improvement of the patient will be long. Improvement will be marked, the reaction of the economy is vigorous, and there is no tendency to any structural change in the vital organs. Any structural change that may be present will be found on the surface, in organs that are not vital; abscesses will form and often glands that can be done without will suppurate in regions that are not important to the life of the patient. Such organic changes are surface changes, and are not like the changes that take place in the liver, in the kidneys, in the heart and in the brain. Make a difference in your mind between organic changes that take place in the organs that are vital, that carry on the work of the economy, and organic changes that take place in structures of the body that are not essential to life. An aggravation quick, short and strong is one that is to be wished for and is followed by quick improvement. Such is the slight aggravation of the symptoms that occurs in the first hours after the remedy in an acute sickness, or during the first few days in a chronic case.

Under the *fourth observation,* you will notice a class of cases wherein you will find very satisfactory cures, where the administration of the remedy is followed by no *aggravation whatever.* There is no organic disease, and no tendency to organic disease. The chronic condition itself to which the remedy is suitable is not of great depth, belongs to the functions of nerves rather than to threatened changes in tissues. You must realize that there are changes in tissues so marked that the vital force is disturbed in flowing through the economy, and yet so slight that man with all of his instruments of precision cannot observe them. Under such circumstances we may have sharp sufferings, but cures may come about without any aggravation. We know then that if there is no aggravation the potency just exactly fitted the case, but here you have a course of things that you need not always expect. Though there is nothing but a true nervous change in the economy after a potency that is not suitable, either too crude, or too high, for that patient, you will have an aggravated state of the symptoms. In cures without any aggravation we know that the potency is suitable, and the remedy, the curative remedy, provided that the symptoms go off and the patient returns to health in an orderly way. It is the highest order of cure in acute affections, yet the physician sometimes will be more satisfied if in the beginning of his prescribing he notices a slight aggravation of the symptoms. The *fourth observation* then relates to cases in which we have no *aggravation, with recovery of patient.*

The *amelioration comes first and the aggravation comes afterwards is the fifth observation.* At times you will see sickly patients, fully as sick as the one I mentioned in the first or second instance, walk into your office and after long study you administer a remedy. The patient comes back in a few days telling you how much better he was immediately after taking the medicine, and now he has three or four days of what appears to be a decided improvement, a prompt action of the remedy. The patient says he is better, and the symptoms seem to be better; but wait, and at the end of a week or four or five days all the symptoms are worse than when he first come to you. It is not a very uncommon thing in severe cases, in case of a good many symptoms, to have an amelioration of the remedy come at once; but whatever you may say, the condition is unfavorable.

Either the remedy was only a superficial remedy, and could only act as a palliative, or the patient was incurable and the remedy was somewhat suitable. One of these two conclusions must be arrived at, and this can only be done by a re-examination of the patient and by finding out whether the symptoms relate to that remedy. Sometimes you will discover that the remedy was an error; a further study of the case shows that the remedy was only similar to the most grievous symptoms, that it did not cover the whole case, that it did not affect the constitutional state of the patient, and then you will see that the patient is an incurable one and the selection was an unfavorable one. It is the best thing for the patient if the symptoms come back exactly as they were, but very often they come back changes, and then you must wait through grievous suffering for the picture; and the patient will wait better if the doctor confesses on the spot that the selection was not what it ought to be, and he hopes to do better next time. It is a strange thing how the patients will have an increase of confidence if the doctor will tell the truth. The acknowledgement of one's own ignorance begets confidence in an intelligent patient.

The higher and highest potencies will act in curable cases a long time. When I say act, I only speak from appearance; I should say they appear to act a long time, for the remedy acts at once and establishes a condition of order upon the patient, after which there is no use in giving medicine. This order will continue a considerable length of time, sometimes several months. The patient will get along just as well without any medicine, and get along better without the medicine that helped him than with it. In curable cases whose prospects are good, they will go along for a long time, and become very much relieved of their symptoms. Now, if the patient comes back at the end of the first, second and third week and says he has done well, that he has been improving all the time from the cm. of *Sulphur,* but at the end of the fourth week he comes back and says. "I have been running down," the physician must then pass judgement. Has this patient done something to spoil the action of this medicine? Has he been on a drink? Has he handled chemicals? Has he been in the fumes of Ammonia? No, he has done none of these things.

This condition is really an unfavorable one. To have a medicine act but a few weeks, whereas it ought to act for months thereafter, will make you suspicious of that patient. If nothing has taken place to interfere with this medicine in his economy you may be suspicious of this case. This *sixth observation is too short relief of symptoms*. The relief after the constitutional remedy does not last long enough, does not last as long as it ought to. If you examine the third observation you find that there you have the quick aggravation followed by long amelioration; but in this, the sixth, you have the amelioration, but of too short duration. In instances where you have an aggravation immediately after, and then a quick rebound, you will never see, absolutely never see, too short an action of that remedy; or, in other words, too short an amelioration of the remedy. If there is a quick rebound, that amelioration should last; if it does not last, it is because of some condition that interferes with the action, of the remedy; it may be unconscious on the part of the patient, or it may be intentional. A quick rebound means everything in the remedy, means that it is well chosen, that the vital economy is in a good state, and if everything goes well, recovery will take place.

In acute cases we may see this too short amelioration of the symptoms; for instance, a dose of medicine given in a most violent inflammation of the brain may remove all the symptoms for an hour, and the remedy have to be repeated, and at the end of that repetition we find only an amelioration of thirty minutes. You may make up your mind, then, that that patient is in a desperate condition; it is too short an amelioration. The action of *Belladonna* in some very acute red-faced conditions is instantaneous. In five minutes I have noticed the amelioration come, but the best kind of an amelioration is that which comes gradually at the end of an hour or two hours, as it is likely to remain. If it is too short an amelioration in acute cases, it is because such high-grade inflammatory action is present that organs are threatened by the rapid processes going on. It is too short amelioration in chronic diseases, it means that there are structural changes and organs are destroyed or being destroyed or in a very precarious condition. These changes cannot always be diagnosed in life, but they are present, and an acute observer, who has been working earnestly for years, will often be able to diagnose the meaning of symptoms without any physical examination whatever, so that he can prophesy as to the patient. Such experiences of an intelligent physician in a family will cause them to look upon him as wiser than anyone else, for he knows all about their constitutions. This he acquires by studying their symptoms, the action of remedies upon them, and their symptoms after the medicines have been given. This enables him to know the reaction of a given patient, whether slow or quick, and how remedies affect each member of that family. This belongs to the physician, and he should be intelligent enough to know something about them when he has been treating them a little while. The old physician is in possession of this knowledge, while the student and the new physician have it all to learn.

Once in a while you will see a *full time amelioration of the symptoms, yet no special relief of the patient,* which is the *seventh observation.* There are certain patients that only gain about so much; there are latent conditions, or latent existing organic conditions, in such patient with fibrinous structural change in certain places, tubercles that have become encysted and lungs capable of doing only limited work, will have symptoms, and these symptoms will be ameliorated from time to time with remedies, but the patient is only curable to a certain extent; he can not go beyond and rise above such a state. Remember this after several medicines have been administered, and the amelioration of the case has existed often the full length of time of the remedies, but the patient has not risen above his own pitch in this length of time. The remedies act favorably, but the patient is not cured, and never can be cured. The patient is palliated in this instance, and it is a suitable palliation for homoeopathic remedies.

Observation eight. Some patients prove every remedy they get patients inclined to be hysterical, overwrought, oversensitive to all things. The patient is said to have an idiosyncrasy to everything and these oversensitive patients are often incurable. You administer a dose of a high potency, and they will go on and prove that medicine, and while under the influence of that medicine they are not under the influence of anything else. It takes possession of them, and acts as a disease does; the remedy has its prodromal period, its period of progress and its period of decline. Such patients are provers, they will prove the highest potencies. When you find a patient that proves everything you give in the higher potencies go back to the 30th and 200th potencies. Such patients are most annoying. You will often cure their acute diseases by giving them the 30th and 200th, and you will relieve their chronic diseases by giving them the 30th, 200th and 500th potencies. Many of them are born with this sensitivity and they will die with it; they are not capable of rising above this over-irritable and over-wrought state. Such oversensitive patients are very useful the homoeopathic physician. After they get out of one proving they are quite ready to repeat it or go into another.

The ninth observation is the action of the medicines upon provers. Healthy provers are always benefited by provings, if they are properly conducted. It is well to be observe carefully the constitutional states of an individual about to become a prover, and to write these down and subtract them from proving. These symptoms will not very commonly appear during the proving; if they do, note the change in them.

The tenth observation relates to new symptoms appearing after the remedy. If a great number of new symptoms appear after the administration of a remedy, the prescription will generally prove an unfavorable one. Now and then the coming of a new symptom will simply be an old symptom coming up that the patient has not observed, and thinks it a new one. The greater the array of new symptoms coming out of the administration of a remedy, the more doubt there is thrown upon the prescription. The probability is, after these new symptoms have passed away, the patient will settle down to the original state and no improvement take place. It did not sustain a true homoeopathic relation.

The eleventh observation is when old symptoms are observed to reappear. In proportion as old symptoms that have long been away return just in that proportion the disease is curable. They have only disappeared because newer ones have come up. It is quite a common thing for old symptoms to appear after the aggravation has come, and hence we see the symptoms disappearing in the reverse order of their coming. Those symptoms that are present subside, and old symptoms keep coming up. The physician must know himself that the patient is on the road to recovery, and it is well to say to the patient that this is encouraging; that diseases get well from above downwards, etc. Old symptoms often come back and go off without any change of medicine. It indicates that the medicine must be let alone. If the old symptoms come back to stay then a repetition of the dose is often necessary.

The twelfth observation. We will notice sometimes that symptoms take the wrong direction. For instance, if you prescribe for rheumatism of the knees or feet, or for a rheumatism of the hands, and relief takes place at once in the rheumatism of the extremities, but the patient is taken down with violent internal distress that settles in the region of the heart, or centers in the spine, you see at once a transference has taken place from circumference to center, and the remedy must be antidoted at once, otherwise structural change will take place in that new site. When diseases go from center to circumference, going out from the centers of life, out from the heart, lungs, brain and spine, out from the interiors, upon the extremities, it is well. So it is that we find most gouty patients get along best when their fingers and toes are in the worst condition. To prescribe for this, and see the heart symptoms grow worse is a most uncomfortable state of affairs, for it is attended with a gradual downward tendency. Eruptions upon the skin and affections in the extremities are good signs. I remember one time I was discharged from a violent old woman with quite a considerable amount of Billingsgate, who told me that when she called me in she could walk about, and now her ankles were swelled up with rheumatism so that she could not move. That patient got another doctor, but soon died. There is a great danger in selecting a remedy on external symptoms alone, *i.e.,* selecting a remedy that corresponds only to the skin and ignoring all the symptoms that the patient may have, ignoring the whole economy and general state of the patient; because it is true that the remedy that is related to the skin alone may drive in that skin disease and cause it to disappear while the patient himself is not cured. Such a patient will remain sick until that eruption comes back again, or locates in another place.

Classroom Notes

Prognosis after Observing the Action of the Remedy

1. Watching, waiting and observing has to be done by the physician in order to judge the changes and then decide what to do and what not to do.
2. What are the changes that we may expect?
    Disappearance, amelioration, aggravation, cropping up of new symptoms and new order of appearance of symptoms are the changes that might happen.
3. The idea should be centered around the patient, whether he is improving or not.
4. The direction that the symptoms take is sufficient to tell us the prognosis.
5. Second appointment should be after three weeks.

Twelve Observations
1. **First Observation**
    A Prolonged aggravation and final decline of patient.
    Interpretation   :   Incurable and doubtful case.
    What to do   :   Decrease Potency Palliate and do not aim at cure.

2. **Second Observation**
    A Prolonged aggravation and final amelioration of patient.

    Interpretation   :   Get the patient before he become incurable but he has a feeble constitution.

| **What to do** | : | Keep him on low potency. Repeat when amelioration tapers off. |

3. **Third Observation**

Short and quick aggravation, followed by rapid improvement.

Interpretation	:	1. Vigorous constitution.
		2. No structural changes except in vital organs.
What to do	:	Ideal reaction, wait. Do not intervene.

4. **Fourth Observation**

No aggravation but recovery of patient.

Interpretation	:	1. Potency exactly fitted.
		2. The condition is not of great depth but only functional.
		3. No organic disease.
What to do	:	Wait. Do not intervene.

5. **Fifth Observation**

First amelioration followed by aggravation.

Interpretation	:	1. The remedy was partially similar.
		2. Obstacle to cure.
		3. The patient was incurable the remedy palliated.
What to do	:	1. Re-examine the case.
		2. You may have prescribed the wrong remedy-give right remedy.
		3. Look for obstacles to cure and remove those obstacles.
		4. If not so then patient is unfavorable. Keep him on palliatives.

6.   **Sixth Observation**

Short relief of symptoms (short amelioration).

Interpretation   :   Blocks to cure.

What to do   :   1. See whether block to cure is unconscious or international. If international ask why?
2. Remove blocks to cure.
3. Administer constitutional remedy in a different potency.

7.   **Seventh Observation**

Full amelioration of symptoms but no relief to patient.

Interpretation   :   1. Patient incurable.
2. Remedy acted as a perfect palliative.

What to do   :   Palliate.

8.   **Eight Observation**

Patient proves every remedy he gets.

Interpretation   :   1. Idiosyncratic patient, over-sensitive patient.
2. Tubercular miasma.
3. Often incurable.

What to do   :   1. Go back to 30th and 200th.
2. Administer inter-current potency of *Tuberculinum.*
3. Good for proving otherwise incurable.

9.   **Ninth Observation**

Action of remedy over provers.

10.   **Tenth Observation**

New symptoms appear after the remedy.

Interpretation	:	Wrong prescription (The greater the array of new symptoms more is the probability that prescription is wrong).
What to do	:	1. Re-examine the case.
		2. Find and prescribe the right remedy, taking in to account totality of the case.

11. Eleventh Observation

Old symptoms reappear.

Interpretation	:	Patient is on road to recovery.
What to do	:	1. Wait and do not intervene.
		2. If the old symptom come back to stay, then a repetition of the dose is necessary.

12. Twelfth Observation

Symptoms take a wrong direction.

Interpretation	:	Wrong remedy.
What to do	:	1. Antidote the remedy.
		2. Try again.

LECTURE XXXVI

The Second Prescription

THE second prescription may be a repetition of the first, or it may be an antidote or a complement; but none of these things can be considered unless the record has been again fully studied, unless the first examination, and all the things that have since arisen, have been carefully restudied that they may be brought again to the mind of the physician. This is one of the difficulties to contend with when patients change doctors, and one of the reasons why patients do not do well after such a change. The strict homoeopathic physician knows the importance of this and will try to ascertain the first prescription. If the former physician is strictly a homoeopathic physician, he is most competent of all others to make the second prescription. It is often a hardship for a patient to fall into the hands of a second doctor, no matter how much Materia Medica he may know. The medicine that has partly cured the case can often finish it, and that medicine should not be changed until there are good reasons for changing it. It is a very common thing for patients to come to me from the hands of good prescribers. I tell them to stay with their own doctor. I do not want them. Such changing is often a detriment to the patient, unless he brings a full record, and this is especially true in relation to a case that has been partially cured, where the remedy has acted properly. If the patient has no reasonable excuse to leave the doctor, it is really a matter of detriment to the patient for a physician to take another's patients at such a moment. It is not so much a question of ethics, it is not so much a question of the relation of one doctor to another because friends can stand all that, but it is only after a tedious inspection of all the symptoms that an intelligent physician is capable of making a second prescription. As a general thing, if the first prescription has been beneficial it ought not to be left until it has done all that it can do. How is the second physician to know that? Then the duty of the physician is first to the patient, and to persuade the patient to return to his first doctor.

The rule is, after the first correction and homoeopathic prescription, the striking features for which that remedy was administered have been removed, a change has come, and the guiding symptoms of the case have been taken out, and only the common and trivial symptoms remain. It is true if the physician would wait long enough, he would see the return of those symptoms, but usually when a patient walks into a doctor's office the doctor is in a hurry to make a prescription and does not wait until the proper time. He at once prescribes on the symptoms that are left, and this is one of the dangers to be avoided, a hurried second prescription. The patients are to be pitied that falls into the hands of such homeopaths. Many patients are wonderfully benefited by the first prescription; they have said to me "Doctor so and so benefited me wonderfully for a while, and then, he did not seem to be able to do me any good." The fact was that the first prescription was a correct one, having been properly chosen, and after that first prescription the doctor administered his medicine so hastily and so indiscriminately that nothing more was accomplished in the case. The trouble was that he did not wait long enough. It makes no difference whether the physician is so extremely conscientious that he does not want to give Sac. Lac., or whether he is so ignorant that he does not know how to give it, the result is the same. The early repetition of the medicine and the continued giving of the same medicine will prevent anything like an opportunity for the making of a second prescription.

If the doctor administers a well-chosen remedy, and repeats it too soon, he never gives the symptoms a chance to come back and call for a second prescription; but they come intermingled with drug symptoms, so that the rational second prescription cannot be made. The second prescription presupposes that the first one has been a correct one, that it has acted, and that it has been let alone. If the first prescription has not acted curatively, or has not been permitted to act the full time, it is impossible to get a second observation. The second observation is made when the case comes to a standstill, for after the first prescription has been made changes occur; there is a coming and going of symptoms, and while these changes are occurring no rational observation can be made of the case; if a second prescription be made during this time, it will be likely to spoil the whole case. If the patient is not given a perfect rest, if medicines are not kept out of the case, we will have no opportunity to make a rational second prescription. But if these precautions are observed, then we can really make an observation upon the return of the original symptoms, which is the first thing to be considered. Perhaps they are not so marked, but that is always the first thing to be looked for, the return of the original symptoms. While the confusion is going on after the administration of the remedy, while internal order is being established in the economy, we do not have the return of the original symptoms. This may be a matter of days, or weeks, or months, but if the return of symptoms is not observed what is there to be done?

Without symptoms what can the homoeopathic physician do? No matter what state the patient is in, what can the physician do without symptoms? There is no earthly guide to the remedy except by signs and symptoms. So that it is the duty of the physician *to wait for the return of the original symptoms.* If the symptoms return somewhat as they were, differing slightly in their intensity, increased or decreased, it is good. If the patient has not had these present symptoms for some time, if there has been a relief caused by the first prescription, and then the symptoms return somewhat as in the original, this is one of the reasons for believing that the first prescription was a good one. If, after an interval of two or more months, the original symptoms return, we need very little information beyond this to know that the first prescription was a good one. In such a case when the symptoms return, when the patient has the same general and particulars as formerly, it means that the first prescription was a good one, that the case is curable, and that the second prescription must be a repetition of the former.

Another reason for making a second prescription is the appearance of a lot of new symptoms taking the place of the old symptoms; the old symptoms do not return, but new symptoms come in their place. The patient says: "Well, doctor, you have cured me of those symptoms I had, but now I have these." The doctor, after examining carefully these new symptoms, immediately looks up the pathogenesis, and it is possible that he will find these symptoms in the drug that he has administered and then it looks like a proving. He asks the patient if he ever had these symptoms before. "Never to my recollection, doctor." Cross-examine him carefully to see if he is not mistaken, until it seems that they are really new symptoms. If so, the remedy has not acted properly. It was not homoeopathic to the case; and yet it was an unfortunate prescription, because it has caused the disease to progress in another direction, developing another group of symptoms. This coming up of new symptoms means that they must be *antidoted,* if it is possible. The new symptoms combining with the old ones must be again studied and the second remedy must correspond more particularly to the new than to the old. It may cause the new symptoms to disappear and possibly have an effect upon the old ones. Any subsequent prescription takes into account all the things that have preceded it, all the conditions that have arisen, and, the third, fourth, fifth or sixth prescriptions have the same difficulties to surmount that are to be surmounted in the second. If the first prescription was an unfortunate one, then all the others are made with difficulty and fear.

It is rarely the case that a new prescription become necessary when the case merely comes to a standstill. The first prescription has been made and the symptoms commence to change in an orderly way; they change and interchange and new symptoms come up, but finally the symptoms go back to their original state, not marked enough to be of any importance, without any special suffering to the patient, and the patient has arrived at a state of standstill. The patient says, "I have no symptoms, yet I am not improving; I seemed to have come to a standstill position." He says this as to himself, not as to the symptoms. He has come to a standstill.

It is the duty of the physician then to wait, and wait a long time, but if after many months no outward symptoms have appeared, no external tendency of the disease, it is true that another dose of the same medicine will not do harm and the same remedy is the only one that can be considered. A new one cannot be entertained, because there is no guide to it; but another dose of the same medicine can cause the patient to be jogged along the way of feeling better, but there should never be any haste about it. Wait a long time when patient come to a standstill; but when, as in the first instance, the return of the original symptoms is observed, then you have some guide to the administration of the medicine.

The second prescription, then, technically speaking, is the prescription after the one that has acted. You may administer a dozen remedies without having any effect upon the economy, and yet no prescription has been administered that has been specific. You may fool away much time in administering remedies that are not related to the case. The result is the same. Consider the first prescription the one that has acted, that one has effected changes, and subsequent to that the next prescription is the second.

The next thing we have to consider *is the change of the remedy* in a second prescription. Under what circumstances must we change the remedy? One instance I have mentioned, when striking new symptoms appear, and there is an entire change of base in the symptoms, so that the headache, perhaps, which has lasted a long time, disappears. After the administration of the medicine, when a new group of symptoms appears somewhere in the body relative to the patient, such as the patient has never had, this new group of symptoms means that a new remedy must be considered, and under such circumstances the change of the remedy will be the second prescription, and the second prescription in this case calls for a change of remedy.

We will suppose another instance where the remedy must be changed. A patient has been for years under treatment for a constitutional chronic disorder, and you have gone through the potencies ranging from the lowest to the highest, and they have acted curatively. You have administered the different potencies, repeating the same potency until it would not act any longer, and then going higher, until you have gone through the whole range of potencies. You can repeat that remedy many times on a paucity of symptoms, when you cannot give another remedy, simply because it has demonstrated itself to be the patient's constitutional remedy. This remedy should not be changed so long as the curative action can be maintained. Even if the symptoms have been changed do not change the remedy, provided the patient has continuously improved. If the patient says he has improved continuously, and though it would be impossible for you, at this date, from the present symptoms, to select that remedy, hold on to that remedy, so long as you can secure improvement and good from it, though the symptoms have changed. Many physicians say: "If the symptoms change, I change the remedy." That is one of the most detrimental things that can be done. Change the remedy if the symptoms have changed, providing the patient has not improved; but if the patient has improved, though the symptoms have changed, continue that remedy so long as the patient improves.

Very often the patients are giving forth symptoms long forgotten. The patient has not heard them, or has not felt them because he has become accustomed to them, like the ticking or the striking of the clock on the wall. Many of the symptoms that appear, and the slightest changes that occur, are old symptoms coming back. The patient is not always able to say that they are old symptoms returning, but finally the daughter or somebody in the house will delight you by saying that her mother had these things years ago and she has forgotten them. This is likely to be the case whenever a patient is proving. So long as curative action can be obtained, and even though the symptoms have changed, provided the patient is improving, hands off. Whenever in doubt, wait. It is a rule after you have gone through a series of potencies, never to leave that remedy until one or more dose of a higher potency has been given and tested. But when this dose of a higher potency has been given and tested, without effect, that is the only means you have of knowing that this remedy has done all the good it can for this patient and that a change is necessary.

There is another instance to be spoken of, and that is when the second prescription becomes a complementary one. A second prescription is sometimes necessary to complement the former and this is always a change of remedy. Suppose a little four or five year old child, a large-headed, bright, blue-eyed boy, is subject to taking cold, and every cold settles in the head with flushed face and throbbing carotids, etc., you say give him *Belladonna* and *Bell.* Relieves, but it does not act as a constitutional remedy. He continues to have these headaches, which are due to a psoric constitution, and the time comes when *Bell.* will not relieve them; but upon a through study of the case, you find that when his symptoms are not acute, when he does not have this cold and fever, he does not have the headache and you see an entirely different remedy indicated. You study over the flabby muscles, and you find his glands are enlarged; that he takes cold with every change in the weather, like enough he craves eggs, and you decide that the case calls for *Calcarea carbonica.* The fact that *Bell.* was so closely related to him and only acted as a palliative further emphasizes it. It is a loss of time to treat more than the first or second acute paroxysm. Do not give *Calcarea carbonica* during the paroxysm, but after the wire edge has been rubbed off by *Bell.,* give him that constitutional remedy that is complementary to *Bell.,* which is *Calcarea carbonica.* Many remedies associate after this fashion.

Then there are series of remedies, as, for instance, *Sulphur Calcarea carbonica* and *Lycopodium clavatum.* A medicine always leads to one of its own cognates, and we find that the cognates are closely related to each other, like *Sepia officinalis* and *Nux vomica.* A bilious fever in a *Sepia officinalis* constitution is likely to call for *Nux vomica,* and as soon as that bilious fever or remittent fever has subsided the symptoms of *Sepia officinalis* come out immediately, showing the complementary relation of *Nux vonica* and *Sepia officinalis.* If the patient has been under the influence of *Sepia* some time, and comes down with some acute inflammatory attack, he is very likely to run towards *Nux vomica* or another of its cognates. The whole Materia Medica abounds with these complementary and cognate relationship.

The second prescription also takes into consideration the change of plan of treatment. The plan of treatment consists in assuming that the case is a psoric one, if looming up before the eyes, all the symptoms in the case and its history indicate psora. The treatment has probably consisted of *Sulphur, Graphites* and such medicines as are well-known to be anti-psorics. The symptoms have run to these remedies; but behold, after you have made the patient wonderfully well, and you have effected marked changes in his system, so that the psoric symptoms have disappeared, he comes into your office with an ulcerated sore throat, with dreadful head pains and with the constitutional state and appearance that will lead you to say, "My dear sir, did you ever have syphilis?" "Yes, twenty or thirty years ago, and it was cured with Mercury." Now, the psoric condition has been subdued and this old syphilitic condition has come up. This, then indicates a second prescription. You have to adjust your remedies to an entirely new state of things. So it is also with regard to sycosis; these states may alternate with each other. When one is uppermost, the other is quiet, so you have to change your plan of treatment according to the state of the patient.

No prescription can be made for any patient except after a careful and prolonged study of the case, to know what it promises in the symptoms, and everything that has existed previously. That is the important thing. Always restudy your cases. Do not administer a medicine without knowing the constitution of the patient, because it is a hazardous and dangerous thing to do.

Classroom Notes

The Second Prescription

The second prescription may be:

    (a)   No prescription (placebo);

    (b)   Repetition;

    (c)   Antidote; and

    (d)   Compliment.

1. Medicine that has partly cured the case can often finish it and medicines should not be changed until there is good reason for changing them. Wait long enough and don't be in a hurry to prescribe.

2. *If old symptoms return* it means the first prescription was a good one. This case is curable. Second prescription if and when needed, must be a repetition.

3. *If new symptom crop up:* then the first prescription was a bad one. It must be antidoted. To antidote, repertoirize combining new symptoms with old ones. The second remedy must correspond particularly to the new than to old symptoms.

4. *If the remedy fails to act, think:*

    (a)   Was the remedy wrong or were you being too clever?

    (b)   Did the patient take his remedy, if not then why?

    (c)   Are there blocks to cure?

5. Under which circumstances do we change the remedy?

    (a)   When striking new symptoms appear and there is an entire change of base (Miasma shifts) in the symptoms.

    (b)   Change the remedy when symptoms have changed but the patient has not improved.

    (c)   Change the remedy when entire range of potency of the previous one is exhausted, and the patient comes to a standstill.

    (d)   A second prescription is sometimes necessary to complement the former and this is always done with a change of remedy. For example *Belladonna* in acute paroxysm and *Calcarea Carb* when paroxysm has subsided. This is called **Serial Prescribing.**

(e)   The second prescription also takes in consideration a change of plan of treatment. This is called **Layered Prescribing.** After the first prescription has addressed one miasma and has subdued it, an underlying second miasma may come up and this may require another class of remedies as a second prescription.

LECTURE XXXVII
Difficult and Incurable Cases—Palliation

WHILE homoeopathy itself is a perfect science, its truth is only partially known. The truth itself relates to the Divine, the knowledge relates to man. It will require a long time before physicians become genuine masters in this truth. In Switzerland the children have been raised for centuries to the knowledge that it is necessary to make watches perfectly, they have been raised, as it were, in the watch factories. Now, when homoeopathy is hundreds of years old, and little ones grow up into the knowledge of it and observe and practice it, our successor will acquire knowledge that we do not posses now. Things will grow brighter as minds are brought together and men think harmoniously. The more we keep together the better, and the more we think as one the better. It is a pity that differences should arise among us when we have so perfect a truth to bind us together.

It is very rarely the case that among the provings of our remedies not one is to ht found which corresponds to the characteristic features of a case. It was rarely so in Hahnemann's day, and it is certainly very rarely the case with our voluminous Materia Medica. Beginners, of course, are obliged to rely very largely upon the repertories. This one thing you can depend upon, the image of the patient's illness becomes more simple when you have done your best to prescribe one remedy after another. In these difficult cases, when you have zigzagged the patient for a number of years, you will find his symptoms become more definite and striking and more clearly understood. Sometimes when I have worked patiently upon a patient for a long time, and I have given several remedies, and the patient has partially improved, she has become disappointed and run off to somebody else, but would come back again and say I had done more for her than anyone else and she would try again. I have found in such instances that time has done much, and that I had little trouble then to grasp the case and make rapid progress. In addition to that, she comes back with a patient state of mind, which is more helpful to the physician than to her. The confidence of the patient helps the physician to find the right remedy. His mind works much better when he feels he is trusted; the confidence of the patient sharpens his intelligence.

Closely analogues to these cases are what may be called alternating complaints and one-sided complaints, those that show but one side. It is not uncommon for a patient's malady to have two sides - one side being manifested when the other side is not. Eye symptoms may be present when the stomach symptoms are absent. You may find that *Euphrasia officinalis* is more sharply related to the eye symptoms that the antipsoric that fits the whole case, and that *Pulsatilla nigricans* fits the stomach symptoms much better than the antipsoric that fits the whole case, but remember that there is one antipsoric that is more similar to the whole patient than these special remedies, because it is better fitted to the generals. The oftener you prescribe for different groups of symptoms the worse it is for your patient, because it tends to rivet the constitutional state upon the patient and to make him incurable. Do not prescribe until you have found the remedy that is similar to the whole case, even although it is clear in your mind that one remedy may be more similar to one particular group of symptoms and another remedy to another group. Very often a remedy that will go to the very center and restore order to the economy will cause quite a turmoil. These alternating and one-sided complaints are sometimes dreadful to manage, and when everything is thrown to the surface or the extremities, e.g., when gouty and rheumatic symptoms have an outward tendency, the patient will run off and leave you.

Incurable complaints - and you meet many - will trouble any physician. The allopath has the means of putting the patients under the influence of strong drugs and making them imagine that something is being done to their benefit, whereas injury is being done whenever they are patched up by strong drugs. It is unaccountable, therefore, that some of our homoeopathic practitioners make use of palliatives that are so detrimental to the patient.

The physician who applies the single remedy in potentized form under the Law of Cure any length of time will easily be convinced that there is no other way of palliation that holds out any permanent hope for the patient. Opium will sometimes relieve pain, stop diarrhœa, and mitigate cough, but woe to the patient. It so annuls reaction that there is no possible development of the symptoms that are necessary to indicate what homoeopathic remedy the patient needs, and while the pain is stopped the patient is not cured. What has been said of Opium is as true of all drugs given to relieve pain. When an opiate must be given, let it be clearly understood that a cure of this patient is abandoned. What thoughtful physician will abandon the hope of a cure during painful sicknesses so long as life endures. In consumption and cancer and wasting sickness the remedy that is most similar to the painful groups of symptoms will ever give the most relief and it is a forlorn hope that tempts its abandonment.

Classroom Notes

Palliation of Difficult and Incurable Cases

1. Alternating and one-sided conditions are dreadful to manage.
2. Try to come up with one remedy that addresses different groups of symptoms.
3. In advanced cases of tuberculosis, cancer and wasting sickness, the remedy that is most similar to the painful group of symptoms will always give the most relief.

LECTURE XXXVIII

Essentials of Successful Repertorisation

A PHYSICIAN must study Homeopathic principles until he learns what it is in the sickness that has to be cured. He must study the Materia Medica until he learns what it is in the remedy that is curative. He must also study the repertory until he learns how to use it so that he finds what he wants when he needs it. The physician must read the repertory rubrics over and over in order to learn what is in it and how symptoms are expressed? It must be admitted that many do mechanical work and fail to realize that repertorisation of any other kind is possible.

The other type of repertorisation is the artistic repertorisation. The artistic prescriber sees much in the proving that cannot be retained in the repertory, where everything must be sacrificed for the alphabetical system. The artistic prescriber must study Materia Medica for long and earnestly to enable him fix in his mind sick images.

I have often known the intuitive prescriber to attempt to explain a so-called marvelous cure by saying "I cannot quite say how I have come to give that remedy but it resembled the sick". We have all heard, felt, and seen it but who can attempt to explain it?

It is something that belongs not to the novice. It is only the growth of art in a scientific mind. This art comes gradually to the experienced scientific prescriber.

This art belongs to the healing artist. If carried too far it becomes a fatal mistake and must therefore be corrected by repertory work done even in the most mechanical manner. The more a physician restrains a tendency to carelessness in prescribing the wiser he becomes in artistic affects and Materia Medica work. Thus repertorisation and Materia Medica must go hand in hand and must be kept in high degree of balance or loose methods and habits will destroy any good worker.

The Value of Temperaments and Constitutions in repetorising

Of late it has become common for Homeopathic physicians to say too much about the *temperament* and *constitution* when analyzing a case.

The mental state of the patient furnishes the most important guiding symptoms, and has nothing to do with the temperament. If by temperament we mean that which is his normal condition, it is an error to include it in the totality of symptoms used as the basis of repertorisation and prescription.

It is a fatal error to confuse what is natural and what is morbid. The Totality is the complex of all that is morbid, and not what is physiological. Always remember, *"The true basis for a Homeopathic remedy is the collection of signs and symptoms, and these must be morbid".*

It is also a fatal error to attempt to classify constitution as an aid to prescribing. The classification of constitution is never useful to the Homeopathic when searching for a remedy. To a genuine Homeopathic physician no two constitutions are sufficiently similar. *Individualization* is the aim of every Homeopathic physician. The symptoms that represent the morbid constitution or disorder of the individual are the ones that a skillful prescriber seeks. Since the classification of constitution is based on common disease symptoms at best these constitution can guide you to a group of remedies for example in Hydro-nitrogenoid constitution anti-sycotic remedies are found to be most commonly indicated but it does not mean that anti-psorics cannot be used even if they fit it the totality of the case. I have been convinced for long that it is bad practice to allow the make up of a patient to suggest a remedy.

A remedy can be selected only after a careful repertorization of every morbid and peculiar symptom in the case. Then will appear in the physician's mind a symptom image which is the true image of sickness, or a sick person, and in that image will be seen the remedy if the symptoms have been compared individually and collectively with the symptoms that are found in the Materia Medica.

The corner-stone of good reportorization is, good and full history taking. The aim of full case taking is to establish totality and individuality of the case.

Individuality of a disease must be known. Such information is best acquired by observation of the multitude of symptomology. One must remember the individuality of the sick manifests itself by peculiar symptoms.

The beginner should not attempt to abbreviate the anamnesis, but should write out full general rubrics and then he must observe. He must also remember that frank pathology will not be a guide to totality. The symptoms expressive of the whole state that existed prior to the cellular change are the things to look for. It is out of this pre-existing state, from which the pathology evolves. Therefore we must observe the language of the symptoms in order to interpet the expression of the cause.

As Homeopathy includes both science and art, repertory work can also be science and art.

The Scientific Repertorisation

The scientific method is the mechanical method, where one first settle the mentals then the physical generals and then see, what are remedies that come up, compare them to the particulars of the patient and choose the remedy after going through the Materia Medica.

The symptoms which are general and particular with the common left out, are always strange, rare and peculiar and therefore characteristic. To collect these is the only way to secure a firm basis for a scientific repertorisation.

The Artistic Repertorisation

The artistic method of repertorisation is an extension of the scientific but it omits the mechanical way. This is a better way but all are not prepared to use it. The artistic method demands that judgment be passed on all mental symptoms and a view to be taken of the general symptoms, after the case has been taken most carefully.

For example if we select the rubric industrious for repertory work then it is not such persons as were born that way but those who have become industrious. That is to say an individual who has been ordinarily industrious, but who develops abnormal urge for work and in this abnormal industrious state he works almost night and day, now this is a sick state. So if we use industrious rubric for repertory work it does not mean an ordinary industrious state but the one that is exaggerated into a symptom.

(**Author's note:* At this point if you will like to know why such an abnormal state exists in the sick individual you would enter the realm of causes and this may change the view of the case.)

The great aim of the Homeopathic physician is to study the representation until the image of sick individual stands out in bold, not the disease type, but the individual with the disease. This can be done by categorizing symptoms into:

1. Peculiar Symptoms

Hahnemann's teachings have never been improved upon. We must be guided by the symptoms that are *Strange, Rare* and *Peculiar*, but how shall we do this?

By first fixing our mind to the symptoms that are common, it would be easy for us to discover symptoms that are uncommon or in other words Strange, Rare and Peculiar. When the common symptoms have been deleted in any given case what remains in uncommon. These Strange, Rare and *Peculiar* symptoms are always predicated of the patient. However some of these common symptoms may become peculiar.

For example: weakness is common if constant but if it comes

only before menses, or before stool, or during a storm, it is at once quite uncommon and worthy of note. These special aggravations are of great help but such observations are often lacking in cases and the generals must be pressed for use.

2. General Symptoms

There are two types of generals, the mental generals and the physical generals.

(a) *The mental generals* are composed of reasoning power, loves, hates and memory. These are of highest importance.

(b) *Physical generals* are the general body symptoms and their circumstances (modalities), such as worse from cold, from warmth, from weather, wet or dry, from motion or rest, time of day etc. Those too are very important because they apply to the whole body.

3. Modalities

Two sets of aggravations/ ameliorations come into view, viz: which apply to the whole man and those which apply to his parts. These are often opposite in parts (organs) from those which exist in general body states of the patient, and they must be looked up in the repertory.

If we do not consider these circumstances (modalities) we do injustice to the patient and his parts. Therefore the circumstances that relate to the general bodily states and the circumstances that relate to the parts/organs must be considered separately, or the view of a given case will be vastly changed.

4. Totality of symptoms

The symptoms of the organs and the parts taken separately give an imperfect or one-sided view of the case. They fail to give the symptoms of the patient in such a form as to present a perfect view. If prescribing is to be made easy, it is to be done by securing such a perfect view of the whole case as will be expressed by saying that *"The sole basis of Homeopathic prescription is the totality of morbid signs and symptoms"*.

5. Key Note Symptom

The task of taking the totality is often a most difficult one. It is sometimes possible to abbreviate the repertory work by selecting one symptom that is very peculiar containing the key to the case. A neophyte cannot detect this peculiarity, and he should seldom attempt it.

The symptoms must be judged as to their value and characteristics, in relation to the patient. The symptoms must be passed in review by the rational mind to determine those that are Strange, *Rare and Peculiar.*

It is often convenient for the experienced to start with key rubric and then take a group of three or four essentials in a given case, making a summary of these and eliminating all remedies not found in all the essential symptoms. But what shall we do when we find several peculiarities in the same patient and one remedy does not cover them all?

Here is where an astute physician will pick up the repertory and commence the search for a remedy most similar to all, by doing the scientific repertorisation.

The success of repertorisation (and that of successful prescribing) depends only upon the view taken of the totality of the symptoms.

To be able to view the totality of symptoms so that, the most similar remedy will appear to the mind is the aim of repertorisation of all healing artists. As the views vary, so varies the success.

———————

Lecture XXXIX

Essentials of Successful Prescribing

PRESCRIBING *the Homeopathic remedy is such a matter of growth and progress that it may be said that the best of the wine is saved for the last.*

It is well to hope and for all that with experience each may attain the high degree of perfection in healing that Hahnemann attained. Much can be done now what Hahnemann could not do, because we have a greater number of remedies, and a greater number of potencies and higher potencies. It is doubtful if the technique of prescribing has made much progress since Hahnemann. It is this direction that all need to meditate. If we will make progress, we must dwell upon the teaching of the Organon

1. We must dwell long upon what it is in the human being that must be changed in order to restore man from sickness to health.

2. We must meditate long upon what it is in remedies or drugs that constitute healing power or principle.

3. At last the physician must know how to adjust the former to the later in order to gain the ends of healing.

Whoever has thought that the medicinal virtues of drugs might be developed in an infinite series of degrees by means of triturating and shaking of the raw material?

—Hahnemann, Chronic Disease.

This opens up the consideration of '*Series in Degrees*', which is the most important subject in treatment of chronic disease.

Whatever potency a physician uses, that single potency is not sufficient for chronic disease. It will generally do for acute sickness. Many chronic sicknesses are cured by keeping the patient under the influence of the one indicated remedy for two or more years. But this cannot be done, with a single potency. Unless the doctrine of series in degree is fully understood, one cannot learn the way to use potencies.

As there are "*Octaves*" of musical tones, so there are octaves in simple substances, through which it is possible to correspond with the various planes of the interior organism of an individual.

Whenever the similimum is found the remedy will act curatively in a series of potencies. If the remedy is only partially similar new remedy will be called for. Many chronic cases will require a series of carefully selected remedies to affect a cure. If the remedy is only partially similar. Though the ideal prescribing is to find that remedy similar enough to hold the case through a full series up to the highest potency.

Observations Regarding the Selection of Potency

There is wonderful latitude between the tinctures and the CM's. In my judgment the selection of the best potency is matter of experience and observation. It is not yet a matter of law.

There is almost an endless field here for speculation and observation but there are also possibilities of bringing out certain rules for guidance as under:

1. The various potencies are more or less related to individuals and it is the individual that we should study.
2. We might well begin with Hahnemann's statement that the 30C is low enough to begin with.
3. Constitution of the individual makes a difference. Some patients are very sensitive to the highest potencies and are cured mildly and permanently by the use of the 200C or 1000C. There are other individuals who are torn to pieces by the use of highest potencies.

4.   Some very sensitive patients will do well in a high potency if they have been prepared for it by the use of lower one.

5.   Nature of the disease makes a difference. Patients with organic disease of heart, lungs, kidney and liver in advanced stage are apt to have their sufferings increased and end hastened by the highest potencies. So is the case with advanced cancers. These cases do better under the 30C or 200C.

6.   It is better to begin with low potency and go higher and higher.

7.   To suit all degrees of sensitivity in chronic diseases the physician must have at his command his deep acting medicines in the 30C, 200C, 1000C, 10M, 50M, CM, DM & MM, potencies made carefully on the centesimal scale. The physician who knows how to use various potencies has ten times advantage over the one who always uses single potency, no matter what that potency is.

8.   In acute disease 1M and 10M are the most useful.

9.   In 30C to the 10M will be found those curative powers most useful in very sensitive women, children and to some men. In sensitive women and children it is well to begin with 30C or 200C at first, permitting it to act as long as it will cause the patient to improve in a generally way, after which the 1M may be used in a similar way. After improvement with that ceases, 10M may be required.

10. From 10M to MM may be used in ordinary chronic disease in persons not so sensitive. (Stoic individual).

The Administration of Remedy

1.   It never matters whether the remedy is given in water, in spoonful doses or given in a few pellets dry on the tongue- the result is the same.

2.   It has been supposed by some, that by giving in one or two small pellets, a milder effect will be secured, but this is a deception. The action or power of one pellet, if it acts at all,

is as great as ten. If a few pellets be dissolved in water and the water is given by the teaspoonful, each teaspoonful will act as powerfully as the whole of the powder if given at once.

3.   When medicines is given at interval, the curative power is increased. This is safe provided the medicine is discontinued with judgment. If a positive effect has been obtained the medicine should always be discontinued. Therefore, it is not always the technical single dose that is the best practice, but the single cumulative effect can always be sought.

4.   In chronic disease for the first prescription the single dose dry on the tongue will be found the best.

5.   The correct observer will soon learn whether the best effect is to be secured by a single dose or a series of doses. After the best effort has been secured there is no exception to the rule- wait on the remedy.

6.   In severe acute sickness in robust constitutions several doses in quick succession are most useful while the condition is worsening but stop the medicine if the symptoms begin to yield.

7.   In chronic disease, after single doses have been given at long intervals and have acted well but it's action is getting feebler and feebler (and the symptoms still call for that same remedy) a series of doses will show a stronger and deeper action, and this is even true if the potency is given much high.

8.   In chronic disease when the 30C and 200C potencies are used it is much often necessary to give the medicine in water than when using high potency.

9.   Very high potencies seldom require repetition. If clearly indicated those produce a long curative action in chronic cases.

10.   If we give very high potency to the feeble and extremely sensitive, we bring back old complaints and symptoms; too hurriedly, and violently and fail to sustain the curative action long enough to eradicate the underlying miasm.

When to administer the medicine:

1. To avoid the shock or aggravation some give the dose at night, others in the morning but there is no difference.

2. A deep acting chronic remedy should seldom be given in the middle of a paroxysm or an exacerbation.

3. It is necessary to nurse the case on to a fortuitous moment and then give the deep acting chronic remedy. This moment comes when the excitement has past - when there is calm. If it be a menstrual suffering, after menstruation. If it be chronic sick headache, after the headache. If it be a fever, after the paroxysm.

LECTURE XL

Trend of Thought Necessary for Development in Homeopathy

THE STUDY of man as to his nature, as to his life, as to his affections, underlies the true study of Homeopathy. A rationale doctrine of therapeutics begins with the study of the changes wrought in man. We may never ascertain causes, but we may observe changes. A physician highly trained in the art of observation becomes classical in arranging what he observes. It will hardly be disputed that the changes in man's nature, without an ideal natural man, will not be thinkable. Whether we observe the changes wrought in man through his own will, through disease, or through drug proving.

Hahnemann has emphasized on the symptoms of the mind. We see how clearly the master comprehended the importance of the direction of symptoms; the more interior, first (the mind) and the exterior, last (the physical or bodily symptoms).

The only possible way to confirm to the above trend of thought and thereby establish a system of therapeutics is by proving drugs as Hahnemann has taught. We may now see clearly what is to be understood by proving drugs, and we may define it as that conjunction of the given drug force with the vital force of man, whereby a given drug has wrought its impression upon man in a manner to make changes in his vital order, so that his sensations, mental operation's and functions of organs are disturbed. When large enough number of provers have registered sensations, mental changes and disturbed functions so that it may be said of a drug that has effected changes in every organ and parts of man and his mental facilities, then may it be said that it has been proved. Not that all of its symptoms have been brought out, but it has been proved sufficiently for use. In other words its image has been established.

The remedy finds its place in man and then develops its own nature. If it has not in it that can rise up and impress man's internal state, it will not be able to develop these symptoms. Man's image is therefore, in all elements of plant and as an when susceptibility exists in man then the proving may be wrought.

Reflect upon the mental state of a man who has used alcoholic stimulants in great excess for many years. His manhood is gone, he is a constitutional liar, and will deceive in any manner in order to obtain whiskey. It may truly be said that he is but an image of his former self. Indeed every drug is capable of rising in its own peculiar way and making such changes in man as will identify itself in the image of man. There is no disease that does not have its correspondence in the three kingdoms.

It is not generally known that the three kingdoms (The Plant, Animal & Mineral kingdom) exist, as to their interior in the image of man.

These substances of the three kingdoms must be examined. They must be examined by understanding, and the quality of each must be ascertained.

It is neither of the material stone, earth ore, quartz's and mineral salts, nor is it of the colors of plants, leaves, buds and flower, neither of stems and stalks or of the substances used, that the eye should behold. It is not density of Platinum, or the whiteness of Aluminum, or the yellowness of Gold, or the toxic nature of Arsenic that one must turn his thoughts to.

Think of the nutritive wheat, corn and barley used for food, and then of the deadly *Aconite, Belladonna* and fox-glove. While thinking of one group as nutritive and the other as poisonous, we make no progress.

We must observe that all these grow and thrive in the same

atmosphere and in the same soil, and by reflection we realize that the former builds up whereas the later destroys the vital force of man. How can we not conclude that there is some primitive substance, too subtle to see with the external eye that becomes the medium of power? This is the field of action of simple substance and the realm of causes.

I have tried many methods for opening the mind to comprehend explanatory terms, in effort to study simple substance to lead the material brain to the realm of non-material mind. There is a strong tendency to depend on what is gleaned by the senses, but the realm of non-material simple substance must be recognized by reason.

To educate the mind, so as to cause it to think interiorly, requires considerable care and study.

It is necessary to transfer the mind from the concrete to the figurative in order to perceive the character of simple substance. Material substance is fed and treated on the plane of nutrition. The non-material substances work on the plane of disorder and cure.

The plane of disorder (sickness) can be perceived in the following order:

1.   Realm of causes (Non-Material simple substances).
    (a)   Perversions of emotion;
    (b)   Perversion of intelligence;
    (c)   Disturbed / perverted memory; and
    (d)   Perverted physical sensations.

2.   Realm of Ultimates (Material substance):
    (a)   Disturbed functions or disturbed organs.
    (b)   Tissue changes and pathological sensations.

Causative factors that excite each of these six planes are parallel to the perverted states in themselves, in each sphere.

Any physician who can view a sick man in this way from first to the last, will be able to secure evidence that will enable him to adjust Materia Medica so that order is re-established.

To heal the sick, physician must perceive what is disordered in the body. He can perceive this only by viewing the phenomenon of disorder. The physician must think from the things first (causes) to things last (ultimates), including all items in their places, and giving each it's full value in relation to the whole.

As of himself a sick individual must be perceived in a grasp collectively, and mentally analyzed by the measures of excess, defect and of perversion.

Correspondence of organs and direction of cure

Hering first introduced the law of direction of symptoms from within out, from above downward and in reverse order of appearance. This is known as the Hering's law. This does not occur in Hahnemanm's writings.

There is scarcely anything of this law in the literature of Homeopathy, except the observation of symptoms going from above to the extremities, eruption appearing on the skin and discharges from mucus membranes or ulcers appearing upon the legs as internal symptoms disappear.

Let's expand on Hering's "within"

The innermost (within) of man consists of Will, Understanding and Memory and these are extended outwards to the physical organism (without) by the voluntary Principle. Keep this idea in mind when considering the direction of symptoms from innermost to the outermost.

A patient returns after a prescription, say with diarrhea. We know it may be elimination. He thinks that he is worse because by his reasoning something has appeared, which he did not have before. Now the doctor will be temped to change the remedy if he is not aware with the correspondence of organs. By his knowledge of Correspondence of Organs he is able to know whether the patient is better or worse.

The physical organs correspond to internal man.

The Understanding (*Intellectual part of an Individual*)

The intellectual faculties (Understanding) consider a proposition presented, weighing it in the light of things learned to determine whether it be false or true. The memory holds it while it is examined and considered. The intellect distinguishes what is received, separating the true from the false. It retains the true and rejects the false.

Correspond this to the GIT (Stomach & Intestine)

The stomach receives food while the intestine digests and assimilates that which is good for the body and cast of that which is not suitable. So the gastro-intestinal tract does to food, what understanding (intellect) does for man.

Similarly kidney do to blood and lungs do to the air we inhale, what understanding (intellect) does for a man.

The Will (*The Emotional part of an Individual*)

The will corresponds to the heart, liver and the sexual organs.

When an individual is sick in Understanding, his rationality is lost and if he is sick in the will, his loves are turned to hate, he desires to destroy his own life or flees from or hates his own children. This disturbance follows the perversion of entire voluntary system.

Through familiarity with Swedenborg, I have found correspondences. With all I have learned in the past thirty years, familiarity with them aids in determining the effect of prescriptions. A man, sick in his mind, does not appreciate how sick he is, and is not able to judge his condition. He thinks he is worse when liver symptoms appear. He says he is worse. That is the course from within to without and thus be not deceived. The threatened condition of liver will pass away with the remedy selected for the mental plane.

These things must be clear or you must take the low plane in Homeopathic art, otherwise you will interfere with your own work, meddling with good work accomplished by the low plane of Homeopathic art. Without such knowledge, knowledge of Homeopathic Materia Medica is insufficient except for acute cases. Homeopathy is suited to old chronic suppressed conditions. Hahnemann did not know correspondence and he did not have time to think over the concept of making of man and he could not develop high potencies (although it seems that with LM potency scale his intent was to go higher than the 30th). Without these no physician can do what Hahnemann said could not be done. He said that effects of drugs are incurable, but you can handle suppressed conditions with this knowledge. Think on these things; meditate and get benefit by these concepts.

The less man knows the less responsibility he has. If you perceive truth, a duty accompanies it. You are a million times more responsible. When you come within range of eternal truth, law and order you take a tremendous responsibility upon yourself.

An Appeal

HOMEOPATHY exists in varying degrees as to application, from the crude with admixture of traditional methods, upto the highest results of absolute obedience to the known law. It is important to avoid thoughts that are destructive to the fundamental principles of Homeopathy.

I desire to have my friends shun some things leading away from Hahnemann's thoughts. True Homeopathy is the object of this Lecture, to maintain the thought and trend of Hahnemann's reasoning.

Every great practitioner admits the value of the law and his efforts to follow it. None of the great prescriber has ever claimed a discovery not fully set forth in the Organon. All in their great accomplishments have said that they based their successes upon the Organon. It is the first book for the student to read, and the last for the old and busy physician to ponder upon.

One of the greatest obstacle to the progress of Homeopathy is found in the minds of its practitioners. The inclination today is to be guided by the personal opinion of men or some man, instead of looking to the principles themselves as authority. The teaching of Hahnemann should not be belittled by the modern opinion of men.

There is too much of a tendency in these days to call attention to the magnitude of our own greatness and our opinion and to create something for men to admire and worship, even if it's only a calf. Men who follow law must recognize Hahnemann's Organon as the fixed and settled authority, and opinion of one or many as of little value.

There is a growing tendency amongst the so-called scientific minds (to explain Homeopathy on the basis of the scientific theory of the day), due to which our young men stand in danger of being drawn into this vortex of ultra scientific confusion.

On the other hand the most dangerous manner of perpetuating Homeopathic truth is to mix it with mysticism. There are some things about this art of healing that pertains to the scientific, of which not one is more important than the proven drug. In no way can we perpetuate our philosophy but by adhering to the proven drug in all our discussions.

It is better to rule out all the fragmentary guess work and makes every report show its relation between drug and disease in the manner designated in our philosophy. By thorough and careful work we will someday complete a Materia Medica whose every symptom will have been repeatedly verified. Then indeed will our art become exact science. Such is the end for which we must labour.

Excerpts from An Address
Preliminary to the study of Homeopathics
By J.T. Kent

Index

V

W